LIFE AFTER TRAUMA

LIFE AFTER TRAUMA

A WORKBOOK FOR HEALING

Dena Rosenbloom, PhD and Mary Beth Williams, PhD
with Barbara E. Watkins

THE GUILFORD PRESS
New York   London

Printed in the United States of America
This book is printed on acid-free paper.

Last digit is print number: 9 8 7 6 5 4 3 2 1

Library of Congress Cataloging-in-Publication
data is available from the Publisher.
ISBN 1-57230-239-9

To my family, friends, and clients; your courage, kindness,
and resilience continually rekindle my hope.
—DR

To Danny Lee King who never lost his will to fight and did not
"go gentle into that dark night" on July 23, 1998.

To my children, Cary, Kirstin, Ryan, and Seth and to
Anastasia and Honey—lives cut short. We love you.
—MBW

CONTENTS

$\mathcal{F}$OREWORD

There are very few self-help resources for survivors of traumatic life events. While researchers and clinicians have developed a literature for professionals, less has been made available to lay readers seeking information about psychological trauma. *Life After Trauma* was written to fill this need. It offers a solid base of understanding and specific tools for the process of healing. "Recovery," "healing," "getting on with one's life," "making meaning," "transforming pain"—these words and phrases suggest hope for survivors of traumatic life experiences. They also require enormous effort—a courage that requires facing terror, enduring shame, and risking connections. For trauma survivors, the effort may seem overwhelming or terrifying, the hope too distant.

This workbook is intended to honor the effort, the terror, and the hope of survivors. Drs. Dena Rosenbloom and Mary Beth Williams are clinical psychologists who have walked through the terror with trauma survivor clients for well over a decade. Their combined research and clinical experience has provided them with an understanding of many elements of recovery. Both have served as gentle guides to people in distress. Both have lent their hearts, heads, and hands to survivors who have risked hope, effort, terror, shame, and connection in order to create a new reality that includes, but is not dominated by, a traumatic past. Readers will be comforted by the gentle, supportive tone of the workbook. The authors' consistent respect for the process of healing allows the reader to approach difficult issues with a feeling of support and connection.

Life After Trauma includes a wealth of information about common responses to horrific events. Readers will find many of their difficulties illuminated in these pages and be comforted to see that others share the painful and confusing feelings and experiences that otherwise might be endured alone. They will find hope in understanding that the most painful adaptations represent heroic efforts to survive and thrive. While honoring survivors' commonalities, the workbook equally acknowledges the uniqueness of each individual. Each survivor has his or her own story and his or her own coping strategies. The authors' extensive experience doing psychotherapy with survivors is evident in the care they take along the way. Readers are guided and encouraged to take care of their needs, to notice their feelings, and to stay connected to the present. The workbook takes a present rather than past focus, and in doing so, helps the reader stay out of dangerous terrain in past memories. Concepts are nicely illustrated and illuminated by a number of straightforward examples.

The core of the book is the examination of five basic psychological needs: safety, trust, control, esteem, and intimacy. In our research and clinical work at the Traumatic Stress Institute (TSI/CAAP), we have found that these needs are highly sensitive to disruptions through traumatic life experiences. Our own clinical experience shows that understanding and changing one's beliefs about these needs can be a very powerful part of healing from trauma. At TSI/CAAP, where Dr. Rosenbloom practiced for over five years, we have found that a focus on the five needs offers survivors hope and tools for healing. The possibilities for healing include stronger relationships with others, an increased sense of connection with oneself, and an ability to disengage from the traumatic past.

As one of the authors of constructivist self-development theory, I am thrilled to see this important part of the theory made more accessible to survivors. In my relationships with Dena Rosenbloom and Mary Beth Williams, I have been impressed by their commitment and sensitivity to survivors, and their understanding of the complexities inherent in the healing process. I thank them for this workbook; I believe it can make a difference in the lives of survivors.

LAURIE ANNE PEARLMAN, PHD
Traumatic Stress Institute/
Center for Adult & Adolescent Psychotherapy
South Windsor, Connecticut

$\mathcal{A}$CKNOWLEDGMENTS

The only way a book such as this can be written is by pooling the contributions of many people. First and foremost, I thank the many clients I have seen over the years, whose commitment to healing has taught me much of what I most treasure and use in my work. I only hope I add to the lives of my clients as much as they enrich mine. Some clients have made direct contributions to this workbook, and countless others have informed my thinking by sharing their struggles and healing process. Each client contributes to my thinking and my work. I can never thank them enough for what they have given me.

I also want to thank my coauthor, Mary Beth Williams for initiating this project. I had thought for several years about embarking on a workbook such as this, but it was her initiative and vision that brought it to fruition.

Many friends and colleagues also supported my efforts. I want to thank Pamela Deiter, PhD, Sandra Hartdagen, PhD, and Sherri Nelson Fitts, PhD. for their generosity in reading the manuscript, giving feedback, and supporting me through our personal and professional relationships. Others who read parts of the manuscript at various stages, offering feedback, support, and valued friendship were Mary Hostetler Hoyt and Marge Hawley. My close friend, Robin Grant Hall, although not directly involved in this project, has also been an invaluable source of support to me in so many ways over the years. I also want to thank Karen Saakvitne, PhD for providing a safe place over a six-year period to talk about my clinical work from week to week. I learned immensely from her clinical sensitivity, compassion and acumen. Even though we no longer meet, much of the wisdom in her words and our conversations returns to me as I need it. My other former colleagues and friends at The Traumatic Stress Institute, Mark Hall, PhD, Amy Ehrlich Charney, PhD, Sarah Gamble, PhD, Dan Abrahamson, PhD, Anne Pratt, PhD, Richard Nicastro, PhD, Molly Beaudoin, and Susan Kupec, offered a community unique in its provision of both intellectual and emotional riches. Brenda Shaw responded to an invitation I presented to a number of trauma survivors to make contributions or proofread the manuscript and provide feedback. She has been extraordinarily generous, spending countless hours providing detailed and carefully considered comments and giving of herself completely to the process of "doing" the workbook. Her level of involvement and commitment has been a testament to the healing and hope possible for people who go through extraordinarily difficult life experiences. I also want to thank Laurie Pearlman, PhD. Not only did she originally cocreate (with Lisa McCann, PhD) the theory upon which this workbook is based (constructivist self-development theory), but she has also been a treasured colleague and kindred spirit since we first met over eight years ago. I look forward to many more years of friendship. My parents, Cordelia and Joseph Rosenbloom, also provided me with support throughout this process. They both read an early version of the manuscript and offered encouragement and helpful ideas. My father's own writing over the years has been an inspiration to me. And my parents' love and devotion have given me a foundation that carries me through my day-to-day life. I am saddened only that my mother did not survive to celebrate the completion of this workbook with me.

I want to extend special gratitude to Barbara Watkins, our editor from Guilford Press. Her tireless work, commitment, excitement, and belief in the project truly made it possible to create a finished and, I hope, extremely helpful resource for trauma survivors. I'm not sure Barbara, Mary Beth, or I knew exactly what we were getting into at the outset of the project, but Barbara's involvement was instrumental in bringing it to the point of completion.

And in a category all their own, I want to thank Matt and Aaron, who keep my life full of joy, hope, challenge, perspective, growth, and comfort. Thank you.

DENA ROSENBLOOM

In 1988, as I began my dissertation, I discovered an article by Lisa McCann, Laurie Anne Pearlman, and others. From that article, I created a 31-item belief scale (The McPearl) that 531 survivors of sexual abuse completed. As I worked with survivors, I learned more of the centrality of their beliefs. In fact, as a conclusion from my dissertation research, I learned that the most significant variable leading to long-term posttraumatic impact of child sexual abuse was the *perception* of the abuse as harmful and negative. From my research on the theory grew the dream to create a workbook that would directly help survivors. This is the final product. I want to thank Dena Rosenbloom for her dedication and patience and Barbara Watkins for her effort and endurance.

I do not have an organization to acknowledge, but I do want to thank those who have supported me during this process—my children, Joyce Braak, MD, Hedi Fried, John F. Sommer Jr., Dr. David Niles, and Lasse Nurmi. Thank you all.

MARY BETH WILLIAMS

$\mathcal{B}$EFORE YOU BEGIN

IS THIS BOOK FOR YOU?

Have you experienced any of the following:

- the sudden or untimely death of a close friend or relative
- being diagnosed with a serious illness
- surviving a natural disaster
- being in a serious accident such as a car or plane crash
- experiencing physical or emotional abuse in childhood or in adult relationships
- being a victim of crime such as robbery, mugging, rape, or drive-by shooting
- seeing the effects of violence in your home or neighborhood

These events can be traumatic when they contradict your understanding of how things are "supposed" to be, and why things happen in the world. They can disrupt your sense of yourself and others. They can shatter illusions about how safe the world really is and how much control you have in your life. When trauma is caused by another person, it can undermine a basic sense of trust in other people; it can make intimacy with others diffi-

1

cult; and it can disrupt your own sense of self-worth and self-esteem. If you have had any of these, or similar, experiences this book can help you.

We are psychologists with specialized training in helping people rebuild their lives after trauma, whether the experiences occurred long ago or more recently. We are involved in psychotherapy, research, and educational programs, all focused primarily on what people need as they heal following one or more traumatic events. We have found that, for many people—whether immediately following a trauma or years later—the following help a great deal: finding comfort, learning to take care of yourself, getting acquainted with who you are now, getting support from others, having information such as you will find in this book, and finding other resources such as those in this book's appendixes. This book is an effort to offer widely information that can most help following trauma.

This workbook is written so you can use it on your own at home. If you wish, it can also be used as part of the psychotherapy process, but not everyone needs psychotherapy following a traumatic event. If you are already in psychotherapy and want your therapist's support in using the workbook, please give your therapist a copy of the "Letter to Mental Health Professionals" that appears at the end of this book in Appendix C. It offers guidelines and suggestions for how a psychotherapist might best work with you as you use this workbook. If you need more help than this workbook can offer, we encourage you to seek a psychotherapist with specialized training in treating trauma. Appendix B offers a list of resources to help you.

HOW THIS WORKBOOK CAN HELP YOU

This workbook is based on the ideas of Lisa McCann and Laurie Anne Pearlman. They looked at the research and professional literature on trauma and gathered information from colleagues and from their own work with trauma survivors. They came to believe that trauma affects us by undermining five basic human needs. These are:

- The need to be safe
- The need to trust

- The need to feel some control over one's life
- The need to feel of value
- The need to feel close to others

When these basic needs are met, we have a psychological cushion to help us cope with life's troubles. When met, these five needs function as buffers, protecting us through difficult times. After trauma, however, you may feel as though this cushion is gone. Suddenly things that were once manageable leave you feeling overwhelmed and unable to cope. You may feel uncertain how to meet your most basic needs or how to get through the day.

> ❈ *Donna, a single woman of 27, saw the world as generally safe as long as she took some minor precautions. Then one day she returned from work to find her home ransacked. Valuable items were missing. As Donna confronted her wrecked apartment she felt her sense of the world suddenly shift. She thought, "I'm not even safe in my own home. I don't have any control over what happens to me."*

Donna can feel safe again although it may not be the same sense of safety and control she had before. She can again have some control in her life. She does not have to live always in fear and distrust. Even when it feels that the worst has happened, it is possible to feel good again. Your reactions to your present day-to-day life are based on the larger lessons that you drew from all your experiences, including the trauma. You believe these lessons to be true—but they may not be and they may be causing their own problems. Has trauma changed your ability to feel safe, to trust, to have self-worth, to be in control, and to be close to others? The premise of this workbook is that traum disrupts you when it changes a basic belief you have about safety, trust, self-worth, control, and intimacy. For example, to believe you can *always* act in ways that keep you safe or in control is an illusion. But it is just as much of an illusion to belief these things are *never* possible. This book's aim is to help you find the real middle ground between always and never, where you can live a more comfortable life. In this book, we want to help you collect and weigh as much evidence as you can and then decide for yourself what you believe.

**Please Read
IMPORTANT!**

This book is designed to help you cope in your present day-to-day life following trauma. The exercises in this book ask you to think about your life right now, *since* the trauma. We do *not* ask you to think about the trauma itself or its details. Please do not use a traumatic situation for any of the exercises in this book. We will frequently remind you of this. Despite our efforts, however, some of the stories and exercises in this book may call up powerful unpleasant memories of your trauma accompanied by overwhelming feelings. One of the first tasks of this workbook is to teach you how to protect yourself should this book trigger overwhelming trauma memories. We begin to do that later in this prologue. For this reason, we ask you to read through this prologue and the first four chapters of this book in sequence. Don't skip ahead until you are sure you have ways to take care of yourself when strong feelings arise.

HOW THIS WORKBOOK IS ORGANIZED

What wound did ever heal but by degrees?
—Shakespeare, *Othello*

The long-term purpose of this book is to help you recover a sense of safety, trust, control, self-worth, or intimacy—whichever of these key areas in your life has been disrupted by trauma. For many people, more than one area is affected bt trauma. First, however, you must lay a solid foundation. The first three chapters in this book give you essential information and skills that you need for all the chapters that follow. *Do not skip ahead* in this book. Work through the first three chapters first so you can

- understand you are not crazy, even though you might feel this way following the trauma
- learn and use effective coping and self-care strategies
- acquire the tools to think through your thoughts, feelings, and reactions.

People who have had a traumatic experience, often feel crazy, abnormal, not like they used to. Recognizing how these new feelings, thoughts, or behaviors result from the trauma can help you feel less crazy or out of control. You are not as crazy as you may feel. It is normal for trauma to make people feel abnormal. Research has shown that trauma can affect the way you think, the way your body feels and reacts, your moods and emotions, and the way you behave with other people. In Chapter 1, "After Trauma: Why You Feel Thrown for a Loop," we describe changes that can be normal reactions given a traumatic experience. You may learn that your reactions are not uncommon for people who have been through the trauma.

Although you may not feel it, you probably still have areas of strength and ways of finding comfort. It is valuable to start recognizing these. Chapter 2, "Ways of Coping After Trauma," helps you identify your strengths, recognize your own current ways of coping, and tells you what strategies can help most. It is important that you find and use ways of coping that work for you. This is especially important when you feel overwhelmed, scared, or disoriented. These are times when your need for care is at its highest, but it is also when you are least equipped to start figuring out what you need, let alone how to get it. Later in this prologue we start to suggest ways to care for and comfort yourself. We will continue to offer additional strategies to help you in Chapter 2. It is especially important to have effective strategies for self-care before taking on the work of Chapters 4 through 8. The work you do in these later chapters can help you heal, but it can also be extremely difficult. It can bring up painful recollections and unsettled feelings. Learning first how to take care of yourself not only makes this journey possible, but also helps in other aspects of your life. It is time and energy well spent.

Once you have found ways to care for and comfort yourself, you can begin to think about whether you have changed since the trauma and if so, how. You may react to situations now in ways that surprise you. Chapter 3, "Thinking Things Through," explains how to make sense of your changed reactions. The process begins with learning how to sort out the facts of a situation from your reactions to it. When you react to a situation, you are actually reacting to what you think the facts of the situation mean. Facts cannot be wished away but facts can have more than one meaning. When you look at a lawn chair while the sun is in your eyes, the chair will be back-lit, a dark shape that is difficult to see. If you move around so the sun is at your back, you will be able to see the chair much more clearly. You will then see the chair's color is not a dull black but perhaps a bright blue. You might realize that the chair seat faces toward you rather than away as you first thought. The facts of the chair have not changed, but the way you see the chair has changed. If you have experienced a trauma, it can be like having stared directly at the sun. Even after you look away, the glare seems every-where and prevents you from seeing things clearly. It can keep you from even opening your eyes at all for awhile.

After trauma, you probably see things differently and so you react to them differently. The trauma itself may be over but you drew larger lessons from it. Those lessons about yourself, other people, or the world around you, now shape how you see the facts in your present day-to-day life. The lessons you drew from the trauma may be useful and valuable, but some of them may also be inaccurate and create additional problems and pain for you. The way out of this situation is to pay attention to the facts, think through your reac-tions, identify the lesson or belief you now have, and then weigh the evi-dence on it.

The basic method of this workbook has two main parts. The first is "Thinking Things Through" and the second is "Weighing the Evidence." We have broken these down into smaller steps, and we give you forms and exercises to guide your thinking at each step. The method can be used with any awkward, troubling, or difficult situation you have encountered in your posttrauma daily life. We will warn you frequently that this process is not to be done with a traumatic situation or a trauma memory although some of the beliefs you examine may stem from or be influenced by your traumatic experience.

Steps for Thinking Things Through
- Sort out the facts of what happened
- Sort out the meaning the facts have for you
- Identify the underlying belief
- Evaluate the pros and cons of the belief
- Imagine alternative meanings for the same facts

- Evaluate the pros and cons of the alternative meaning
- Consider how to check the accuracy of these beliefs
- Put the process in perspective

Steps for Weighing the Evidence
- Brainstorm ideas for collecting evidence
- Rank ideas by lowest risk first
- Carry out lowest risk ways to collect evidence
- Record and weigh the evidence for and against the belief

When you feel ready and have self-care and self-comfort activities that work for you, you can begin Chapter 4. This helps you think through the most important basic need: safety. Don't skip over this chapter or move on to the other chapters without first making sure you have tools for feeling and keeping yourself safe.

Chapters 4 to 8 help you think through each of the five needs—safety, trust, control, self-esteem, and intimacy. In each of these chapters we help you think about the meaning of a basic need. If you think each need can only mean one thing, you may be surprised. What do we need when we need safety? What can it mean to trust? Can power mean more than one thing? By what standards can we value ourselves? What do we need when we need intimacy? There are no right or wrong meanings for any of these needs. Meanings are not facts. The important thing is to figure out what *you* need. The goal of this book is to help you find ways to get enough of each of these five needs.

We wrote this book because we believe that healing is possible and well worthwhile. But the work that we invite you to do in this book is difficult and sometimes painful. You might well ask, "Why do this work?" The painful messages about yourself and others that you learned from trauma may hold you back from taking in new messages with more hope and higher accuracy. As Pat Conroy wrote in his novel *Beach Music,* "For me memory was the country of the usable past but now I began to wonder if there was not also a danger to unremembrance. I had recently become acutely aware that mistranslation, mistakes of emphasis, and the inevitability of flawed interpretation of an experience could lead to an imperfect view of things" (p. 402).

Because the work you do with this book can be difficult, it is important to take full advantage of all the ways you can make it easier. The rest of this prologue describes some of the important ways you can do this. These include knowing when to set this book aside, as well as knowing when and how to take care of yourself.

TIPS AND CAUTIONS FOR USING THIS WORKBOOK

Finding Companions: The Comfort of Others

A pleasant companion reduces the length of the journey.
—Publilius Syrus, *Maxims*

Think of yourself as on a healing journey. Much of the work of healing is best done with one or more supportive persons. Trauma is isolating and can leave you feeling disconnected and different from others. Sharing your experiences and feelings, although scary, can help. We encourage you along your way to seek support from friends, family, a therapist, and/or a support group. Opening yourself up to how you think and feel after trauma can be hard work. Saying thoughts and feelings aloud to yourself or someone else can feel frightening or wrong. But the difficulty and the fear are actually natural and normal parts of healing. You may want to retreat at times—take courage and know that struggle is to be expected. The difficult feelings you encounter while doing this work provide opportunities for personal growth and change. But if at any point you feel stuck, or unsure of how to move ahead, we recommend that you find a helping professional who is trained in the treatment of trauma to offer additional support. Guidelines to consider as you look for a therapist are included in Appendix B.

The Importance of Self-Care Strategies

That I feed the beggar, that I forgive an insult, that I love my enemy . . . all these are undoubtedly great virtues. . . . But what if I should discover that the least amongst them all, the poorest of the beggars, the most impudent of all offenders, yea the very fiend himself—that these are within me, and that I myself stand in need of the alms of my own kindness, that I myself am the enemy who must be loved—what then?
—Carl Jung, *Psychology and Religion: West and East*

Healing means attending to and respecting *all parts* of yourself, including the difficult parts of your emotional life. Respecting and listening to your feelings may not come naturally now but can become so with practice. The most difficult feelings are often the most important ones to listen to. Such feelings tell you when you need to care for and comfort yourself; they tell you when you are pressing against the limits of what you can handle; they tell you when you have exceeded those limits. When your feelings give you these messages, we urge you to put this workbook aside and do something special for yourself. *The Woman's Comfort Book* (good for women and men) offers a number of helpful ideas for self-care and self-soothing. This and other publications are detailed in Appendix A at the end of this workbook. Throughout the workbook we have also included relaxation exercises and made other suggestions for calming yourself.

One group of trauma survivors suggested the following ways of calming down when distressed. Try any or all of them. Add more to the list when you think of them.

- Allow yourself to cry, it provides a good release and relief.
- Write in a journal, draw, or use another medium to record your thoughts or feelings.
- Perform a monotonous, routine activity; for example, play solitaire on your computer or do a puzzle.
- Read.
- Rent a movie.
- Spend time outdoors in nature.
- Visualize the distress; put it into an imaginary or real object outside yourself such as a locked box or other container. Containers are designed to hold things.
- Exercise.
- Count to yourself. (It may help to use a watch, your pulse, or objects in the space around you).
- Breathe deeply and fully.
- Hold an object that soothes you, for example, a stuffed animal, rock, or koosh ball.

- Go for a walk.
- Garden.
- Rock in a chair.
- Visualize a safe place; go there in your mind or in reality.
- Listen to music.
- Talk to a friend, family member, therapist, or other safe, trusted person.
- Take a warm bath or shower.
- Discover and participate in an enjoyable hobby.

We suggest that you create and post a list of activities for self-care in a prominent place at home, for example, near your bed or on the refrigerator. The more distressed you become at a given time, the more difficult it can be to take care of yourself. This list can remind you of things that help. The sooner you notice strong or difficult feelings emerging, the easier it will be to calm and comfort yourself.

Make a list now of self-care strategies that have worked for you in the past, or that you imagine could bring you comfort:

∞ My Self-Care Activities

1. _____
   _____

2. _____
   _____

3. _____
   _____

4. _____
   _____

5. _____
   _____

Affirmations and Soothing Self-Talk

An affirmation is a positive statement you say about yourself or others. You say it to yourself either silently or out loud. Affirmations can help you restore a sense of safety, security, and calm. Repeated saying of affirmations can also counteract the effects of negative thoughts that go through your mind, sometimes automatically. Given time, affirmations can help you shift some of your basic ideas about yourself.

Focusing on an affirming thought takes practice; it can be difficult to hear the positive statement over the internal noise of trauma-related thoughts and feelings. This is why we recommend you prepare affirmations ahead of time. Have them ready when you need them. To be effective, affirmations should have the following two qualities: (1) they must be phrased in positive terms and (2) they must be possible.

A positive affirmation is about something you have or can do. A statement about something you *do not want* or *will not allow* is not positive. If it has a "not" in it, it's probably not an affirmation. For example the statement, "I have safe and loving people around me," is an affirmation but the following is not: "I will not let people with whom I feel uncomfortable into my life."

Affirmations must be possible. They must be something you can really imagine operating in your life. For example, if you recently experienced a trauma that has left you feeling totally unsafe, the statement, "I have safe and loving people around me" may be a comforting affirmation of your situation. The statement "I am totally safe, wherever I am" would directly contradict your actual trauma experience. For good reason, it would be difficult to believe and so you would be unlikely to find much comfort in the message. Table P.1 (see next page) gives some examples of negative thoughts and possible affirmations to counter them.

Like an affirmation, soothing self-talk can help you become calm. It is particularly helpful in the face of difficult emotions. Much as a parent soothes a child, or close friends comfort one another, you can learn to speak kindly and gently to yourself. This can also help in times when you feel critical and harsh toward yourself. When Kerri felt overwhelmed by childhood memories of her father's abusing her, she said the following to herself in a gentle way,

I feel like I used to feel, but I am safe now. This is different now. I am safe here. I am safe. My father is very far away. He can't hurt me anymore. I'm big and strong now. I just feel like this because this happens whenever I hear from him. I know I'm safe because I know how to take care of myself now. I'm grown up, and there are people around me who help keep me safe.

In some of the later chapters we will refer again to affirmations and soothing self-talk and how they can help you.

Caution: When to Set the Workbook Aside

It is normal to feel the full spectrum of emotions as you go through this workbook. You may at times feel strong and able to move ahead. At other times, you may feel vulnerable, tired, or anxious. These varying states are a natural part of the healing process. It is important to respect your emotional reactions. You can learn from your feelings.

Throughout this book, we include brief descriptions of trauma survivors' experiences as examples. We believe these can help you better under-

TABLE P.1

Painful Thought	Possible Affirmations
I'm so alone.	I can reach out to others if I choose. There are people who can understand me. I am a part of the world; I belong.
Nobody cares about me.	My {parent/partner/friend} loves me. I am lovable I am a worthwhile person.
Nothing ever works out.	I can get through this. Sometimes things work out.
Something terrible is going to happen.	I'm OK; I'll be OK. I'm safe here and now. I can handle what comes up. The odds are, everything's going to be OK. I can survive and heal from great hardship.

stand how your own trauma experience has affected you. But you may find the examples distressing. If you find this happening, *skip* the examples. You can identify them easily because they are italicized within the text, and set off by the symbol ❧.

Emotions—like the senses of hearing, smell, touch, taste, and sight—offer cues that can keep us safe. If you touch a hot stove, the feeling of pain signals you to pull your hand away quickly. Similarly, if you feel anxious or upset it can also be a cue to pull away. Pay attention to those feelings before you forge ahead with this workbook. Put the workbook aside if you need to. You may need only a brief respite. But other times, you may need more extended periods for a break or self-care. The following is a checklist of warning signs that you might need a break from this workbook.

Caution! If You Have One or More of These Signs, Take a Break from This Workbook

- You begin to have times, or you have more times, when you do not feel completely present in your body or surroundings, or you lose time (also known as dissociation).

- You begin to have flashbacks (images) or more frequent flashbacks of the trauma that intrude into your mind.

- You have feelings that seem unmanageable or flood you.

- You experience irritability, strong anger, depression, fear, anxiety, sadness, or other feelings, particularly if they feel out of control or if you do not understand their source.

- You begin to injure yourself or you injure yourself more frequently (including cutting, scratching, burning, substance abuse).

- You are behaving more compulsively in areas such as eating, working, sexual activity.

- You are completely numb, unable to feel any emotion.

- You have a desire to isolate yourself and avoid others.

- There is a dramatic change in your sleeping or eating patterns.

If you experience any of these signs, step back to consider what you might need, then take care of yourself before continuing in this workbook. For weeks, months, or years following a trauma, you may find that you cannot cope with as much stress you could before. You may now need to take care of yourself at times and in ways that you did not need to before the trauma. This is a common response to trauma that does not reflect poor willpower or weakness; it is a part of the way that traumatic events can change you. The relaxation exercises and other self-care ideas throughout the workbook provide helpful ways to respond to stress.

Coping with Triggers of Past Traumas

Reminders of past experience, whether positive or negative, are called *triggers*. Something in the present triggers a memory of the past. The trigger is often in the form of something you see, hear, taste, or feel. For example, a particular song can suddenly put you back in time with a good friend. But if the triggered memory is of a traumatic event, you may feel afraid, trapped, or helpless. You may feel as if you are back in the traumatic situation.

Reminders of your traumatic experience may be everywhere or only occur occasionally. A car accident victim may flash back to the accident each time she hears tires screeching on a road. An assault victim may suddenly feel back in the midst of the attack when he is unexpectedly approached from behind. The smell of alcohol on someone's breath may remind a victim of her attacker. Emotions themselves can trigger the memory of a past trauma; for example, fearing the loss of an adult relationship can evoke a flood of painful feelings of abandonment related to the loss of a parent long ato. Feelings can quickly bridge you back to a past experience when you felt a similar emotion. This can leave you feeling puzzleed by your strong reaction to a present situation, until you recognize the connection to the past. Often, the connection to the past may not be obvious, and at times you may not be able to figure it out right away. The more you learn about your emotions from the trauma, the easier it will become to know when past emotions get triggered in the present.

Reading this workbook may trigger difficult feelings and memories at times. If this happens, take time out to care for yourself. You may find this difficult to do— *but do it anyway.* Even a trigger that appears to be small or inconsequential can expand rapidly into the big reservoir of feelings associated with the traumatic memory. Paying attention to your feelings and then caring for yourself are the key ways you learn to stop becoming overwhelmed or retraumatized.

Recognizing what things are triggers for which negative feelings puts you in a better position to shift out of the negative feeling state. These are times that self-care strategies can be helpful and you can begin to plan for them in advance. For example, if feelings of fear get triggered, finding ways to feel safer will help.

❖ *When Kerri thought about her abusive father, she often felt terrified. Although he lived several states away, she felt in immediate danger. She was unable to convince herself that he was far away, and she would feel his presence close by.*

Kerri developed the following plan for times when this occurred for her:

Triggers for Fear	Self-Care Plan
Receiving letters from her father	Talk to husband about feelings
	Listen to favorite music
Christmas holidays	Wrap self in comfortable blanket and lie down in bed for a while
	Work on computer (distraction)
	Soothing self-talk
	Call a friend

You can create a self-care plan for your own triggers by answering the following two questions:

1. What events or other experiences trigger bad feelings or memories for you?
2. What self-care strategies would be useful at those times?

Consider your answers, then write these things down in the box headed "My Self-Care Plan for Triggers." Make a copy and put it in an accessible place, such as on your refrigerator or tape it up somewhere in your bedroom.

✤ My Self-Care Plan For Triggers

Triggers	Ways to Self-Care/Self-Comfort
1. _____	_____
	_____
	_____
2. _____	_____
	_____
	_____
3. _____	_____
	_____
	_____

If you are unable to complete this exercise now, feel free to return to it later. While thinking about your experience, and going through the workbook, you are likely to become more aware of how trigger events might apply to you. Add to the list over time as additional triggers and self-care strategies occur to you.

CHAPTER ONE

AFTER TRAUMA: WHY YOU FEEL THROWN FOR A LOOP

TRAUMA: noun; a bodily or mental injury usually caused by an external agent.

TRAUMATIC EVENTS ARE EXTRAORDINARY, not because they occur rarely, but rather because they overwhelm the ordinary human adaptations to life. Unlike commonplace misfortunes, traumatic events generally involve threats to life or bodily integrity, or a close personal encounter with violence or death. They confront human beings with the extremities of helplessness and terror, and evoke the responses of catastrophe. The common denominator of trauma is a feeling of intense fear, helplessness, loss of control, and threat of annihilation.

—Judith Herman, MD, *Trauma and Recovery*

WHAT IS TRAUMA?

What makes an event traumatic? There are two conditions: First, there is the nature of the event itself; it usually involves actual or feared death or serious physical or emotional injury. Second, there is what the event means to the victim. Some experiences, such as combat or rape, are likely to be traumatic for anyone. But other events are experienced as traumatic by one person but not by another. Why? It is because how you experience the event—what it means to you—is just as important as the event itself.

❀ *Paul and Kirk were in similar serious car accidents. Paul is shaken and upset, but over time, life gradually returns to normal. Kirk feels more deeply shaken; his life changes in some fundamental ways. For Paul, the accident was a bad experience; for Kirk, it was traumatic.*

17

There is no "right" or "wrong" reaction to any trauma. In different circumstances or at different times in his life, Paul might experience an event as traumatic but Kirk would not. The particular ways in which people are affected by trauma can widely differ. This large range of differences reflects the normal differences among people.

COMMON REACTIONS TO TRAUMA

There is a tremendous range of frequently occurring reactions to trauma, including the ones that feel "crazy" or unlike anything you've felt before. Some people withdraw into silence; others seek out support or have a pressing need to talk about what happened. Some feel drained of all energy, never getting enough sleep; others are consumed with nervous energy. Some are preoccupied with thoughts about what they could have done differently to prevent what happened; others are filled with anger and rage at the injustice of it all, or feel a deep sense of helplessness.

Each person reacts to trauma in a unique fashion, depending on the particulars of the trauma and the person's unique self and history. Your emotional makeup, personal, family and relationship history, age at the time of the trauma, social and cultural relationships, previous coping strategies, availability of support before, during and following the traumatic experience—all these factors shape the meaning of the event for you. Also shaping your reactions are the particulars of the event such as the degree of violence or the element of surprise. Traumatic events shake the foundation of a person's life. Certain traumatic experiences, such as extremely early experiences of abuse, may interfere with or even prevent a person from developing a solid sense of self. Trauma can affect the whole person, including changes in body, mind, emotions, and behavior. The next section describes some of these common reactions to trauma. They are summarized in Table 1.1.

Physical Reactions

- *Trauma is a major stress and it is common for the body to react.* You may have physical symptoms such as rapid heartbeat, muscle tension, nervousness, and sleep difficulties, or any of the other reactions listed in Table 1.1. Alternatively, your physical reaction may be to feel numb or out-of-touch with your body.

TABLE 1.1 Some Common Reactions to Trauma

Physical Reactions	Mental Reactions	Emotional Reactions	Behavioral Reactions
Nervous energy, jitters, muscle tension	Changes in the way you think about yourself	Fear, inability to feel safe	Becoming withdrawn or isolated from others
Upset stomach		Sadness, grief, depression	Easily startled
Rapid heart rate	Changes in the way you think about the world	Guilt	Avoiding places or situations
Dizziness		Anger, irritability	
Lack of energy, fatigue		Numbness, lack of feelings	Becoming confrontational and aggressive
Teeth grinding	Changes in the way you think about other people	Inability to enjoy anything	Change in eating habits
	Heightened awareness of your surroundings (hypervigilance)	Loss of trust	Loss or gain in weight
		Loss of self-esteem	Restlessness
	Lessened awareness, disconnection from yourself (dissociation)	Feeling helpless	Increase or decrease in sexual activity
		Emotional distance from others	
	Difficulty concentrating	Intense or extreme feelings	
	Poor attention or memory problems	Feeling chronically empty	
	Difficulty making decisions	Blunted, then extreme, feelings	
	Intrusive images		
	Nightmares		

Mental Reactions

• *Changes in the way you think about yourself.* You may have previously thought of yourself as strong and independent, but people who have experienced brutal, unexpected attacks or some other trauma may think they can no longer control their fate. You may now feel much more fearful and vulnerable. Your sense of being in control and able to protect yourself may have been shattered.

• *Changes in how you think about the world.* Some events seem impossible to understand. How can you explain to a six-year-old why her mother and father have been killed in an automobile accident? Why are so many innocent lives lost in repeated terrorist attacks or natural disasters? Tragedies such as these can challenge your basic sense of order in the world.

• *Disruptions in your thoughts.*   Images from the trauma may pop into your mind unannounced and unwanted. You can't seem to stop these images or stop replaying parts of the event over and over in your mind.

• *Confusion in your sense of what happened when.*   You may be uncertain about the order of traumatic events or unclear about certain details of what actually occurred.

• *Heightened awareness of your surroundings (hypervigilance).*   Following some traumatic experiences, you may feel extremely alert and aware of your surroundings. You may scan a room more carefully as you enter to see who's there, where the exits are, and whether there seems to be any risk or danger. You may position yourself near the exit or with your back to the wall. It may be hard to let your guard down and relax.

• *Lessened awareness, disconnection from yourself (dissociation).*   When feelings become overwhelming and there seems no way out of the situation that triggers them, one protective reaction is to cut off the feelings. This can be experienced as "being outside" yourself, as looking at yourself from outside your body, as feeling very spacey and out of touch with your feelings, or as not being aware of what is going on around you. Everyone experiences this to some degree, for example, when you "space out" and don't hear part of what someone is saying to you or when driving, and you suddenly don't remember having reached the next portion of the road. More extreme examples are called *dissociation* and can include not remembering significant or extended portions of your childhood, or finding that there are parts of the present day or week that you do not remember. This is discussed in Chapter 2 when we address dissociation in more detail.

Emotional Reactions

• *Feelings of fear, inability to feel safe.*   A person who has experienced frequent emotional and physical threat continues to feel unsafe, even when circumstances no longer pose a danger. This can include a sense of being unable to protect yourself and feeling unprotected or threatened by others.

- *Loss of trust in yourself or anyone else.* Whether the trauma was a random event or a deliberate action by another person, it can leave a deep sense of distrust. You may feel you cannot count on people or things being a particular way. You may no longer trust your own abilities or judgment.

- *Loss of self-esteem; feeling shame and hate toward yourself.* Survivors of accidents or crimes may feel responsible in some way for causing what happened. If only you had been smarter, quicker, or somehow better, the event would not have occurred. You may feel that because this happened to you, you must have deserved it.

- *Feeling helpless.* Being abused, or caught in a natural disaster, crime, or accident can make us all realize how helpless we can be. In the case of repeated occurrences of trauma or tragedy, you may feel that you are helpless no matter what you do. After experiencing powerful or repeated situations in which you felt helpless, you may come to feel that your actions cannot change or influence current situations. This could leave you feeling especially vulnerable to future harm or devastating loss.

- *Feeling chronically empty.* After going through a traumatic event you may feel empty, used up, and numb, unable to attach any particular name to how you feel.

- *Blunted then extreme feelings.* As a victim of a traumatic event, you may have only dull or numbed feelings of dread, terror, horror, and rage about what happened to you, and you may not feel able to express these feelings. You may then experience sudden and unexpected surges of strong or even overwhelming feelings that are difficult to control.

❀ *After a friend of hers committed suicide, Dawn felt nothing. She knew that she should be feeling sad, confused, or angry, along with the other people who were grieving her friend's death. But she just felt totally shut down and numb. Occasionally, however, she shocked herself when, alone in her car, she became easily angered by other drivers and found herself shouting at them for actions that never bothered her before. The rage she felt at these times seemed out of proportion but the anger just seemed to take over and not let go for some time.*

You may vacillate between these two extremes: At times you may express your emotions when they feel too powerful to contain, or your feelings may simply shut down when you become overwhelmed by their intensity. Generally, you may find it more difficult to manage your feelings.

Behavioral Reactions

- *Becoming withdrawn or isolated from others.*   You may start withdrawing and avoiding other people. There could be many reasons for this, for example, it may feel safer or more comfortable to be alone.

> ❖ *In college, Nancy was date raped by two different men on two separate occasions. She no longer wants to establish any type of relationship with men, let alone date. Nancy is uncomfortable participating in social activities sponsored by her work or her church and spends most of her time alone. Since these assaults, she hasn't been able to develop any new close relationships.*

- *Avoiding places or situations.*   Reminders of the trauma may bring back painful and unpleasant memories. You may find yourself avoiding such reminders even if it means disruptions in your day-to-day life.

> ❖ *Ron had worked and socialized downtown for years, before being assaulted at gunpoint on his way to work one day. Although he was never afraid of being in the city before, he could no longer return to work, or even meet friends or go to the many other favorite evening spots he used to frequent. Being in the city, around all of the familiar sites that used to feel safe, had become vivid reminders of the assault.*

- *Becoming confrontational.* You may find yourself challenging or provoking others. You may pick fights or argue more than before.

- *Changes in eating patterns or other changes in behavior.*   You may find yourself eating more or less than you used to, exercising more or less. You may gain or lose weight as a result. Other behaviors such as sleep patterns or sexual activity can also change.

The above list of common reactions to trauma is by no means complete, but it serves to illustrate the range of possible typical reactions. You may have feelings, thoughts, or experiences that you don't see listed here; this does not mean that your experience is abnormal; it means only that there are too many possible reactions to list them all here.

SUPPORTIVE RELATIONSHIPS CAN CHANGE FOLLOWING TRAUMA

Supportive people are a primary resource for healing after traumatic experiences. But traumatic experiences can challenge and change some or all of your existing relationships. Even when you have supportive friends, family, a partner, or work environment, you may nevertheless feel isolated after trauma. Previously supportive people in your life may not know how to help you. Old friends and family may not be able to understand what you are going through, and this can greatly increase your sense of loss. They may themselves feel scared, confused, frustrated, or helpless. In Box 1.1 (see next page), we offer a list of suggestions for how others can help. You can copy this and give it to whomever you wish. This list may also clarify ways that you can speak with those around you about how they can help.

You may find, however, that some people are uncomfortable with your new, unfamiliar, or even raw feelings, particularly if they are unaccustomed to seeing you that way. Some of their discomfort may reflect their own struggle, feeling unable to comfort you or take away your pain. Sometimes, letting a person know that you understand that they won't be able to take away your pain, but that you need someone to listen to you or hold you, without offering advice, helps caring people better know how to help. Others, even some who care, may still be unable to provide the kind of support you are looking for at various points following the trauma.

You may withdraw from some relationships. You may feel a loss of connection or intimacy in some relationships, even those that you maintain. It is OK to protect yourself from relationships that feel hurtful. We suggest that you try to talk to a friend or family member about your struggle with that relationship before pulling away. For instance, you could say, "I know you care and are really trying to help, but I just need some distance right now." Trying to preserve generally safe and supportive relationships through

BOX 1.1   How Family and Close Friends Can Help Trauma Survivors

If someone you care about has suffered a trauma, you may not know how to help. How do you express your support to someone who is reeling from a traumatic experience? There are things you can do both for yourself and the other person.

1. Having a loved one encounter a threat of physical harm or death can itself be experienced as a trauma. You will have your own reactions to hearing about or seeing what your loved one survived. *Take care of yourself* or you will not be of any help to the survivor. Get support for yourself from others, *not* the survivor. It will be important for you to keep in touch with your own other friends, family members, or supportive people.

2. Get as much information as you can about trauma and its impact. Read or talk to a professional to gain a better understanding of the survivor's reactions.

3. Ask the survivor what you can do to be helpful, and then really try to do it. Everyone's response to trauma is different. Everyone's needs following trauma are different. Try not to assume that you know better than they do what they need.

4. Don't try to fix the person's problems, or make the feelings go away. The survivor is likely to think you are uncomfortable and cannot tolerate his struggle. He may try to conceal his feelings, which may simply create more distance in your relationship.

5. Help the survivor find other support systems, such as a support group, psychotherapy, or relevant professional talks in the community. Or, if you know of someone else who has had a similar experience, you might suggest that speaking with that person might help. You might also mention supportive people in the trauma survivor's existing social network with whom it might be helpful to talk (for example, a trusted friend or family member). Provide suggestions and offer to assist in any way you can, but don't push. Remember number (3) above, and don't assume you know better than he does what he needs.

6. If you do not live with the survivor, try to keep some connection with her, even if it's just an occasional supportive phone call or note.

7. Whenever you can, just *listen*.

8. Try to be patient. Healing from trauma occurs over time and takes time.

difficult times will ultimately serve you well, both through the immediate posttrauma period as well as over the long term.

If you can, try to keep up the connections you have with others in whatever ways feel comfortable or manageable, whether it's an annual holiday card, a phone call, or going to a movie. It does not have to be long conversation over dinner. Just letting others know you appreciate their calls, but aren't up to extended talks or visits, can help keep concerned people within reach until you are ready to reach out. You need to attend to your own needs. But as you will see later in this workbook, connecting with others is a basic need we all share.

CHECKING IN WITH YOURSELF

Reading through the possible posttrauma reactions in this chapter may have stirred uncomfortable feelings for you. Take the time now to "check in" with yourself. How do you feel right now? What do you need? Do you need comfort and a break from this work? If so, what are some of the self-care activities that you listed in the box provided in the prologue? Try doing one of those right now, and come back to the workbook when you feel ready.

Why Check In with Yourself?

When feelings are uncomfortable, it's normal to want them to go away. Trying to ignore discomfort or distress is one way to do this. This solution, however, is only temporary and can cause bigger problems later. Distress can escalate and interfere with your day-to-day activities. Just as it is best to care for a cold so it doesn't turn into pneumonia, it is best to care for emotional distress before it creates bigger disruptions. The first step in reducing emotional distress is to recognize that it's there when it's still fairly mild. It's at this point that you can effectively reduce the distress by caring for yourself. But if you are in the habit of pushing aside or ignoring emotional discomfort, you may not find it easy to notice. This is why, from time-to-time throughout this workbook, we will remind you to do it. Take the time for self-care as you notice the need. Learn to notice on your own when you need self-care and comfort.

How to Check In with Yourself

The ability to notice and recognize emotions is a skill. If noticing mild to moderate feelings of distress is a new skill for you, it will take practice. The more you do it, the better you will get. Box 1.2 lists the key steps for how to check in with yourself. Follow these steps now.

Did you notice any of the emotional or physical reactions described in the box? If so, do you need to find someone to talk to? Would listening to

---

BOX 1.2   How to Check In with Yourself

- Stop whatever you are doing. Be still and silent for a moment.

- Turn your attention to how your body feels.

- Notice any tension you are holding in your body. For example,
    tightness in your shoulders?
    a knot in your stomach?
    clenching of your jaw?
    holding your breath?
    biting your nails?

- Notice any emotions you feel now, or felt while reading. For example, are you feeling:
    upset?
    sad?
    angry?
    lonely?
    frightened?

- Notice if your thoughts are racing or if it is difficult to stay focused.

If you have noticed any of the above emotional or physical reactions

- stop moving ahead in this workbook

- consider what might be helpful in relieving any discomfort *before* moving ahead with the next section of the workbook soothing music be helpful? Would a hot bath help? Or spending time outside, gardening, or taking a walk? Relaxation or massage? Think about what resources might be available to you, or what might be helpful as you do the difficult work of healing.

LEARNING TO RELAX

Relaxation exercises can directly counteract physical tension in your muscles and calm you emotionally. But it is natural for different people to respond in different ways while trying to relax. For example, some trauma survivors feel vulnerable when relaxing, because the exercises typically suggest that you close your eyes and pay attention to internal images and sensations. Be sure to find a safe place where you feel comfortable enough to relax. When first learning to relax, some people have a sensation of floating, light headedness, or some other unexpected feeling. Try to continue relaxing through these feelings. Relaxing, like any other skill, takes practice. As you practice, you will be able to achieve that relaxed state more and more quickly and completely. Stick with it; don't be discouraged if it feels awkward or ineffective at first. This is a normal part of learning. Box 1.3 (beginning on the next page) provides the steps for a useful relaxation exercise.

For most people, relaxation exercises are pleasant or neutral. However, if your traumatic experience included any kind of hypnosis or mind control, emotional invasion or brainwashing, you may want to read through the relaxation exercises before trying them as exercises. If for any reason they don't feel safe or comforting, you may want to modify them in some way, or skip them for now.

If you think it would be helpful, take the time to do the relaxation exercise in Box 1.3 now. First read and try to remember the sequence or speak the script slowly onto an audio tape, which you can replay each time you need to relax. You may also have someone whose voice or presence you find comforting read this onto an audio tape.

BOX 1.3   Relaxation/Visualization Script

This is going to be a time of complete relaxation. Make a conscious effort to relax as totally as possible. Get into a comfortable position and close your eyes. For the next few moments, concentrate on your breathing.

Try to see and feel your lungs, sensing how they feel as you breath in (pause) . . . and feel them as they are completely expanded (pause) . . . and exhale and sense how they feel as you release.

There is no right or wrong way to do what you are doing now. Whatever results you get are perfect results. And if all you do is relax, that is absolutely fine.

This is not a time to worry about any of the things that are happening in your day-to-day life. This is a time only for you. You are in control.

Now, once again, concentrate on your lungs. Picture them in your mind's eye. Inhale and see if you can imagine them filled with strengthening oxygen. And exhale and imagine them as you relax.

If your mind drifts away, and you want to, just bring yourself slowly back to where you are or where you want to be. You are doing nothing wrong, and anything you do will be a success.

And now, in your mind's eye, you can see or hear a message, and the message is RELAX. All over, every cell of every bone, of muscle, nerve, organ and skin tissue, feel a sense of melting into relaxation.

Now, bring your attention to your left foot and ankle, and as you inhale, gently flex your foot, and as you exhale, release and relax your foot.

Now bring your attention to your right foot and ankle, and as you inhale, gently flex your foot, and as you exhale, release and relax your foot.

Let all the cares of the day drain out through your feet.

And any noise you may hear will only deepen your relaxation.

And now, feeling the muscles of your left calf, inhale, contract the muscles of your left calf and exhale and let it relax.

And now, feeling the muscles of your right calf, inhale, contract those muscles, and exhale, letting them completely release.

And, of course, adjust your breathing rhythm to what is most comfortable for you, remembering to inhale relaxation, peace, and love for yourself, and to exhale tension and all the pressures of the day.

This is a learning process . . . learning to relax . . . learning to be at ease . . . learning to be peaceful with yourself.

And now, bring your attention to the muscles of your left thigh, inhale and contract the muscles of your left thigh, and exhale, feeling relaxation pour in.

Bring your attention to the muscles of your right thigh, inhale and contract the muscles of your right thigh, and exhale, feeling release throughout both legs.

And now shift your focus to your behind, inhale and contract your behind, and exhale, letting your bottom relax.

And again, shift your focus to your stomach, inhale and contract your stomach, and exhale and let your stomach relax, relax, relax.

And now, bring your attention to your chest, inhale and feel your chest fill with oxygen. And as you exhale, release any tightness that may be there. Let all the tensions of the day just relax out.

And there's that feeling, that concept of relaxation consciously in your mind and body that is the sensation of relaxation.

Bring your attention to your hands. And as you inhale, close both your hands tightly, and as you exhale, release and let go. Let go of everything you are holding onto and relax.

You may open your palms to receive warmth and vitalizing energy. And feel the sense of relaxation move up through your hands, through your forearms, through your elbows, and up to your shoulders.

And focus attention on your shoulders, and as you inhale, contract your shoulders, hold, and as you exhale, feel all the tension that is there release out.

And feel the point between your shoulders, the base of your neck, and feel warm energy melting away any build up of pressure that is there.

(continued)

BOX 1.3   Relaxation/Visualization Script (continued)

And feel this warm peaceful energy move up through your neck, feel your neck release. Your head is comfortably supported, and your neck relaxes completely.

And the muscles of your face now. Gently tense the muscles of your chin, your mouth, your nose, your cheeks, your eyes, and your forehead, and then let your entire face loosen and relax.

Let yourself be as relaxed as you now are. If there is any part of your body that is not completely relaxed, inhale now, and let any last bit of tension melt out as you exhale.

And if your attention drifts, that's fine, just as long as you are completely comfortable and relaxed.

Many things are changing in your body, all of which are normal and wonderful, just through your relaxation and visualization.

And now, imagine yourself at the top of a flight of 10 steps going down. You have been at the top of the stairs before, and you will be again. So this is completely familiar and feels safe to you. This is a time when you can just put your trust in the world. You may see these stairs as leading deeper into your self, to your inner place of peace and harmony. You will not be out of control in any way. You can trust. And everything is going to turn out exactly as you want it to.

And now, we are going to walk down these 10 steps, and with every step you take, you are going to relax just a little bit more.

And now, if you will, you may take the first step down. And with every step, your relaxation will continue to deepen.

And you may take another step down. And now you've taken two steps down.

And take another step down, relaxing just a little bit more with each step you take down.

And take another step down.

This is a time for relaxation. It is not necessary for you to go to sleep but if you want to that is fine. Or, if your mind drifts away, that's fine. Nothing that you do is wrong.

And so, take another step down. Feel relaxation flow throughout your body.

And now you are halfway down the stairs. You have five more steps to go.

And take another step down. And see yourself on the sixth step and see how comfortable you feel, and how secure you feel and how trusting you feel.

And take another step down. And there is the word RELAX shining right before you.

And take another step down. And you have taken eight steps toward total relaxation.

And take another step, and feel yourself completely release. You have taken nine steps with one more to go.

And now take the last step down, and you are all the way down to the bottom of the stairs. You are at your core of peace and comfort. If you want to, as you remain in a state of complete relaxation, picture yourself before a gently moving stream. The sound of the running water is comforting. And if you can, listen to the sound of the running water. Really try to hear it (pause) . . . tinkling, gurgling, washing the rocks . . . . And the sun is shining down on your body in a way that can't hurt you at all, keeping you toasty warm.

And feel a light breeze over your body and how soothing it is. You can hear the breeze as it moves through the trees, gently rustling their leaves. And hear the stream as it flows over the rocks.

And underneath your feet is the warm earth, and behind you is a rolling meadow, friendly, protective, and full of flowers in bloom. And now, while you are standing there, perhaps you can see yourself at a time when you were very happy, content, and secure. And feel that happiness, feel that security, that carefree feeling, and know that is you. And remember that any noise you hear will just relax you further. And you can call back this feeling of happiness and contentment any time you want to. It is your feeling, your memory. The only one in the world who has that memory is you.

And now, see yourself at the bottom of the same flight of stairs you just came down; you are going to walk back up those stairs. When you reach the top of the stairs, you will open your eyes and be back at the place where you started, feeling completely alert, and at least as well as you felt when you started, and most likely, much better and much more relaxed.

And so take the first step up, take a deep breath in, hold it comfortably, and exhale.

And now, the second step up, still feeling relaxed. And the third step up, and another deep breath in, holding it comfortably, and exhale. And take a fourth step up, continuing to feel very at ease.

(continued)

BOX 1.3   Relaxation/Visualization Script (continued)

And take the fifth step up . . . and you are halfway up . . . take another deep breath in, and exhale as you continue coming back.

And now take the sixth step up, and continue with the seventh step up. Your breathing is even and relaxed.

And take the eighth step up, remembering that when you reach the tenth step, you will be back where you started, feeling completely alert and at least as well as you felt when you started and, most likely, much better. And so, take the ninth step up, with another breath in, and out, and take the tenth and last step up, holding on to your feeling of complete relaxation.

And you are back at the place where you started, feeling completely alert and at least as well as you felt when you started, and most likely, much better. You can open your eyes now, and bring yourself comfortably back. . . .

Modified with permission from a script by Harold H. Benjamin, PhD, creator of the patient active concept ANP, founder of The Wellness Community, an organization providing psychological, social, and emotional support for cancer patients and their families throughout the country. The National Training Center is located at 2716 Ocean Park Boulevard, Suite 1040, Santa Monica, California 90405.

CHAPTER TWO

WAYS OF COPING AFTER THE TRAUMA

COPING: verb; the successful struggle to overcome problems or difficulties.

IF TODAY the situation is not very satisfactory, but you have hope for tomorrow, you can live.

—Suichi Kato

TO WISH to be well is a part of becoming well.

—Seneca, *Theodora*

By "coping" we mean any effort that makes a hardship easier to bear. The hardships we face may be minor, such as getting stuck in traffic, or they may be much more serious, such as a life-threatening accident. For trauma survivors, the hardships can extend beyond the event to the troubling reactions that follow. You may feel it is not possible to go on at times, yet you *are* finding ways to get through the day, the week, the months, and even the years. These are your ways of coping.

People can cope by withdrawing, reaching out, blaming themselves or others, getting information, cleaning, exercising, relaxing, spending time in nature, drinking or using drugs, working, hurting themselves in some way, eating, sleeping, reading, or writing. Some of these coping efforts are clearly helpful, whereas others have drawbacks or are clearly harmful. Some may barely work, if they work now at all, but they continue to be used because at least one time in some context, they worked and made sense. Coping strategies, however, can outlive their usefulness as a situation changes.

In the prologue and Chapter 1, we described some specific ways to help you cope with the challenging feelings that could arise as you read this workbook. In this chapter, we invite you to think about the ways in which you usually cope with difficulties. Most of us learned ways to cope long ago and we may not have thought much about them since. It is quite possible to keep using strategies without realizing that they don't work anymore or that they have significant drawbacks. What do you do in a tight spot? Does it help? Does it have drawbacks? Would you like to find better alternatives?

In this chapter, we also describe ways of coping with stress that have been shown to work well. You may not have used these strategies before, but they could help you now. If you are using them already, it is valuable to recognize that you have resources already that you may not fully appreciate. The coping strategies we focus on in this chapter are primarily ways of managing the most difficult emotions that arise after trauma. You could probably use some immediate strategies for dealing with these feelings. In the next chapter, we explain how thinking things through can be a way of coping. However, it is difficult to think straight when you are overwhelmed by emotion. That is why we first offer some strategies for dealing with your feelings.

TRAUMA CAN DISRUPT HOW YOU COPE

You probably use different strategies for different situations, depending on how much stress you are under, how upset you are, how prepared or caught off-guard, how frightened you feel, or who else is involved. There are many different ways of coping. The more coping skills you have, the better prepared you are to respond to different situations. Coping is like a tool kit filled with different sizes and shapes of tools, each designed for its own specific purpose. If one tool does not work well, it is good to be able to reach back in the box for another. Just as a hammer is not the best tool for all jobs, the same coping strategy will not work well in all situations. In fact, there are a number of jobs in which a hammer would result in more damage than repairs. Even so, a person will tend to use and reuse the same general sorts of coping strategies.

When a person tends to rely on the same strategies for a range of different situations, this becomes a pattern of coping. In a situation as minor as a traffic jam, some people will honk, yell, or change lanes looking for a faster way. Others will use the time to listen to music or books on tape. Still others will make phone calls or just think. These patterns of coping, also called *coping styles,* can be vastly different for different people. Yet for each person, there is often a typical pattern. Approaching problems directly is one kind of pattern, whereas avoiding difficult issues for as long as possible is another. Other particular coping styles include tending to reach out to people for support; tending to pull away from others; making quick decisions and taking immediate action; taking a long time to consider options and weigh a decision. Despite coping patterns and preferences, most people can be fairly flexible in responding to the stresses and strains of everyday life. But the greater the stress, the more likely people are to fall back on what is most familiar.

❧ *Dorothy's typical way of coping was to reach out to friends. She called friends when she felt down, needed advice, or wanted company. She was ecstatic when she finally got pregnant after trying for a long time. She immediately called several of her closest friends to share the good news. She talked to them about all the details, from the physical changes she was going through, to her ideas for naming the baby. Dorothy was devastated when she had a miscarriage four months into the pregnancy. Again, she called her closest friends to tell them the sad news. She was extremely upset for a long time after, but she found comfort in her friends' kind words, caring, and willingness to talk about what happened.*

Dorothy's existing style of coping worked for her when she most needed it. Reaching out to others for support is often a helpful way to cope with stress. Other ways of coping, however, work well in some areas of life but not so well in others.

❧ *Everyone saw Valerie as a very independent, "do it yourself" kind of woman. Her friends and coworkers admired her willingness to hold an opinion different from everyone else's and to fight for what she believed in. The problem was that no one really felt like they knew her; she never joined them for casual time going out for drinks after work or seeing a movie on the weekend. She spent most of her personal time working at home. When her mother unexpectedly died, Valerie took two weeks off from work and then returned to her normal work schedule. She never spoke with anyone about what happened or how she felt. She seemed okay but behind closed doors at home, she spent all her time in bed. She didn't shower or dress on the weekends, and she didn't answer concerned calls and notes from friends. She felt overwhelmed with sadness, loss, and loneliness, but she could not make herself reach out for the comfort that others wanted so much to offer.*

Valerie's independent coping style served her well at work but she did not know how to get emotional support when she most needed it. As for so many people, Valerie believed that "coping" meant always being able to handle something by herself. She thought that if she couldn't deal with a difficulty on her own, something must be wrong with her. The truth is that everyone, at some time, needs help from other people. It is normal to need help. Life is hard. Coping, in large part, is knowing when you need support, assistance, or care, and then knowing how or from whom you can get it. Sometimes ways of coping that worked very well before trauma suddenly stop working afterward.

❋ *After Sandy's car accident, she felt jumpy and anxious much of the time. The things she used to find comforting—taking hot baths or reading novels— didn't seem to offer relief anymore. She had to learn new ways of comforting herself. She tried several alternatives before finding the ones that work for her now. She discovered that more physically active strategies, such as taking a walk or doing yoga, are more effective now.*

Coping can become even more difficult after a trauma when one need, such as the need for safety, gets in the way of meeting other needs.

❋ *Clara was a sophomore in college and frequently went out with friends. One evening, she was returning to her dormitory from a night class when she was sexually assaulted by a stranger. After that, she no longer felt safe going out after dark. This meant that she spent far less time with her friends and started feeling quite isolated. She became limited by her fear and this cut off access to one of the main resources that previously helped her cope with day-to-day stress: her friends.*

No one should have to choose between two or more basic needs, such as being safe and having close friends. But traumatic experiences and their aftermath can seem to put you in just such a situation, in which there is no clear or simple solution. When trauma makes it more difficult to get any basic need met—for safety, control, trust, self-esteem, or intimacy—its impact compounds, making things increasingly difficult over time. For Sandy, a first step to feeling better was to recognize that her way of coping had a big drawback. There were better alternatives. How are you managing to get through your day? Does it have long-term costs? Do you wish you had other ways to make your life easier? If you haven't considered these questions before, you can do so now. The next section will help you do this.

IDENTIFYING YOUR WAYS OF COPING

The following is a list of coping strategies. It was created by the authors after speaking with survivors of a wide range of traumatic experiences. The items include a variety of ways that the survivors tried to cope. Some methods are helpful, some outdated, some created new and different problems.

Go through the checklist and put a check mark next to any item that describes how you reacted, even once, to a difficult situation, whether minor or major. For instance, what did you do last time you had an upsetting fight or disagreement with someone close to you? If the item is a way you *regularly* react, put two checks. Remember not to use your traumatic experience as an example but, rather, other day-to-day situations that arise for you. Once you have gone through the list, look at the questions that follow. These will help you think about what you do to cope.

Ways I Cope: Checklist

_____ I confront the situation head on.

_____ I distance myself from the situation.

_____ I distance myself from myself.

_____ I control myself.

_____ I use relaxation techniques.

_____ I escape through dissociation or forgetting.

_____ I escape through abusing alcohol or other drugs (including prescription drugs).

_____ I act to take care of things myself.

____ I become very aware of the needs and emotions of others.

____ I learn or develop special skills.

____ I call a friend.

____ I call a supportive family member.

____ I call an unsupportive friend or family member.

____ I keep on trying and trying and trying.

____ I become very tolerant.

____ I try to get all the facts.

____ I imagine the worst possible ending.

____ I debate things within myself.

____ I try to see the situation as positive.

____ I see myself as bad.

____ I see myself as a failure.

____ I shame myself.

____ I accept responsibility when appropriate.

____ I create appropriate boundaries with other people.

____ I create rigid boundaries.

____ I give up my boundaries.

____ I use fantasy to escape.

____ I sleep.

____ I become totally involved in taking care of someone else, not myself.

____ I play down the seriousness of what is happening (minimize).

____ I try to earn forgiveness for wrongdoing.

____ I show a sense of humor.

____ I do something creative.

____ I turn to a higher source of wisdom (this could involve another person, a book, or a Higher Power).

____ I dream.

____ I trap myself.

____ I make do with what I have.

____ I plan.

____ I watch television.

____ I overwork.

____ I do busywork.

____ I educate myself.

____ I abuse others.

____ I neglect myself (poor diet, little exercise).

____ I hold onto rigid or irrational beliefs.

____ I find a physical release (walk, swim).

____ I repeatedly hurt myself.

____ I self-mutilate.

____ I make suicidal threats or gestures.

____ I attempt suicide.

____ I do art work.

____ I write in a journal.

____ I work at a hobby.

____ I find a mission.

____ I seek out a social situation.

____ I talk with others about what happened.

____ I find someone who will listen to me.

____ I seek out emotional support.

____ I find help to complete certain tasks.

____ I find help with problem solving.

____ I help others.

____ I just don't think about it.

____ I deny the impact of the event.

____ I deny that the event even happened.

____ I lose sight of the facts.

____ I learn more about what happened.

____ I blame myself.

____ I split into alternate selves.

____ I involve myself in daily tasks.

____ I avoid daily tasks.

____ I lie.

____ I manipulate.

____ I overcontrol myself.

____ I lay guilt trips on others.

____ I don't sleep.

____ I overcontrol my environment.

____ I create chaos around me.

____ I become perfectionistic.

____ I do criminal or illegal acts.

____ I see the world in a negative light.

____ I act in ways so others will see me negatively.

____ I turn to my Higher Power.

____ I turn to the safest person I know.

____ I identify the sources of my fear.

____ I express my anger without hurting myself or others.

____ I become enraged and express anger in ways that can be hurtful or harmful to myself or others.

____ I become addicted to relationships.

____ I become overdependent.

____ I develop a compulsive behavior.

____ I develop an obsession.

____ I do things to excess.

____ I pray.

____ I seek out others who have experienced the same thing.

____ I go to therapy.

____ I join a support group.

____ I remind myself that things could be worse.

____ I look for any sense of meaning that will help explain what happened.

____ I decide I just won't be bothered by what happened.

Thinking about Your Coping Strategies

Go through the list again and look at the items you checked. If helpful, write them down on a separate piece of paper. The ones you checked twice are the strategies you use most when in difficult situations. For each item checked, ask yourself:

- Does this strategy work? Does doing this, in any way, make the situation easier? If it doesn't work, perhaps it is time to look for alternatives.

- If the way of coping works, does it have negative sides? Is there a cost to using this strategy? How high is the cost? Could there be less-costly alternatives?

- When does the strategy work best? Does it always work or only sometimes? Before, during, or after a difficult situation arises? At any or all of these times? Perhaps a strategy will work best in one kind of situation but not others, or at a specific time but not others. Knowing this can help you determine when or when not to use a strategy. It is important to recognize the ways your coping strategies work well for you, appreciating your strengths. We don't want you to forget what you are doing well when you focus on what you hope to change.

Think about all the items with two checks. Can you see any patterns? Do the items tend to match any of the following general coping styles:

Do you tend to take action, face things head on, and try to solve problems?

Do you tend to talk to somebody when you have difficulties?

Do you tend to lie low, avoiding or distancing yourself from problems?

Do you tend to keep difficulties to yourself?

Do you tend to choose strategies with harmful consequences?

Think about your ways of coping as you read the next section.

GUIDELINES FOR COPING EFFECTIVELY WITH STRESS

As we mentioned earlier, not all ways of coping are as effective as others for a specific person, in a specific situation. In some situations, the choices for how to cope might be very limited. When people do have choices, however, research has shown that there are some ways of coping that consistently work better than others for most people. The availability of supportive people has been found to be one of the most valuable buffers before, during, and following stressful events or stretches of time. Box 2.1 lists 10 strategies that have been shown to reduce the stress that accompanies change. These guidelines also help more generally to prevent, reduce, and manage stress.

The stress of trauma can make many of the 10 effective guidelines for coping seem impossible. For example, by itself trauma can make people less

---

BOX 2.1   10 Effective Ways to Cope with Stress

1. Be flexible, try new things, experiment.

2. Learn all you can about what is going to happen.

3. Plan ahead.

4. Avoid impulsive changes.

5. Try not to change too many things at once, especially when you are under stress.

6. Pay attention to your reactions and feelings.

7. Talk to others who have survived similar changes or experiences.

8. Seek support from people who can listen, offer feedback, or help in other ways.

9. Allow yourself to grieve any losses that accompany the change; try not to downplay, minimize, or otherwise discount the impact on you. Even positive changes may have aspects of loss.

10. Take your time.

Adapted from S. W. Osgood, *Abandon Yourself*. Washington, DC: National Institutes of Health, 1978.

flexible. But by reading this book, you are already trying something new. You may have more flexibility than you realize. Reading this book is also a way of "learning all you can" about trauma, how it has affected you, and what you can begin to do about it. Notice that these guidelines also say that sometimes the best way to move forward is to move slowly. "Take your time" means that it can be good to lie low for a while. The 10 effective ways of coping are woven throughout this book. Consider them your basic tool kit.

In the rest of this chapter, we talk about two areas where trauma can cause very stressful changes. First, trauma can disrupt your relationship with yourself. This includes how you think and feel about yourself and how you treat yourself. A changed relationship with yourself can result in floods of extremely difficult, unpleasant feelings. Feeling good about yourself makes it easier to face many of life's challenges. But feeling bad about yourself makes everything harder, including taking care of yourself. The next section talks about how to cope with negative feelings.

A second difficult stress after trauma can be changes in how you think and act in the world and with other people. These changes can sometimes put you at risk for further harm and trauma. However, there are things you can do to manage hardship in both these areas, as we discuss further on in the section "Staying Safe out in the World."

COPING WITH NEGATIVE FEELINGS

The emotional impact of trauma can be devastating. Your emotions may feel unbearable, even toxic. Two feelings in particular can follow traumatic events and feel overwhelming—self-hatred and shame. These feelings may be a direct result of what you have been told about your worth. They may result from being treated disrespectfully or from being repeatedly abused, discounted, ignored, or humiliated.

At the time of the trauma you may not have had control over what happened or how you felt. At times, it may still feel that way, even though what happened is actually now in the past. The danger may be gone, but it may not always feel that way. You can shift your physical and emotional state by, first, reminding yourself that you are in a different time and place from when you experienced trauma initially. You probably have greater choice and control now than you did then. Second, find ways to comfort and soothe your-self. We have provided ideas for doing this throughout the book, such as re-laxation exercises. You may not think they can be much help, but consider this: It is not possible to be tense and completely relaxed at the same time. Learning to relax will directly relieve your tension and anxiety, even if for brief periods initially. Learning to relax can help you feel more in control as well as calmer. The feelings you learn to evoke through self-care and self-comforting exercises are, in many ways, the opposite of those evoked by the trauma. You can learn to use them to help counter and manage negative feel-ings that now seem out of your control.

Knowing How to Comfort Yourself

Comforting yourself is at the top of our recommended list for coping with negative feelings. Finding ways to do this may have been easy for you before the trauma; perhaps those techniques still work. If they don't work anymore or if you never had effective ways to self-comfort, try to find some now that will work for you. Have you tried any of the self-care tips in the prologue? You don't have to wait until you are upset to try one; in fact, that is the hard-est time to try something new. Try a new way to self-comfort now. Examples can include therapy, fantasy, drawing, friends, exercise, nature, hugs in safe relationships, creating more order in your physical space or routine. There are endless possibilities, and you will likely add to the list over time. If it is difficult for you to think about how to take care of yourself, consider what you would say or do for a friend in a similar circumstance. Then do that for yourself. A new golden rule could read: *Do for yourself as you would do for others*.

Can you now list three ways to self-comfort that work for you?

_____

_____

_____

You can use your answers as a plan for what to do when negative feelings threaten to overwhelm you. If you made a list of self-care activities in the prologue, you can use those activities in the same way.

If you cannot yet list self-comfort methods that you know work for you, consider putting this book aside while you find and practice some strategies. Managing feelings can be difficult when the feelings are painful, frightening, or overwhelming. Reading this workbook could trigger such feelings. Before you go further in this book, it is important that you can protect yourself by having ways to cope with powerful feelings.

For some people, harming themselves brings a kind of comfort. If this is true for you, try not to judge yourself for this, but do begin to consider and experiment with other ways to self-comfort. Try just one, perhaps a relaxation exercise, or listening to some of your favorite music. Any new strategy might take some practice before it works well. Stick with it if you believe it could be helpful and is not harming you. If you are concerned about harming yourself, we suggest that you consult a therapist who is familiar with the aftereffects of trauma. We also recommend the excellent book by Dusty Miller, *Women Who Hurt Themselves*. More information on both is given in the appendices. Seeking support and resources from other people is one of the 10 effective guidelines for coping with stress. This is what many other people do to cope, and it works. You don't have to tough it out alone. But when you do have ways to comfort yourself, the next step is knowing *when* to use them.

Knowing When to Self-Comfort: Paying Attention to Your Feelings and Reactions

Self-comforting can stop negative feelings from getting more intense; it can also lessen the intensity. But to do this, you need to pay attention to your feelings and reactions. This is one of the 10 recommended ways of coping with stress listed earlier. If you can allow yourself to notice negative feelings *before* they become overwhelming, you have an opportunity to keep them from getting worse. In Chapter 1, we explained how you can begin paying attention with the exercise, "How to Check In with Yourself" (p. 26). The earlier you notice discomfort building, the sooner you can act to comfort yourself. This is, however, easier said than done.

When feelings are especially negative and uncomfortable, most people do not want to pay attention to them. Trying not to pay attention is, in fact, a coping strategy that can help, for short periods of time. Did you notice the following coping strategies on the checklist you just completed: "use fantasy to escape," "decide I just won't be bothered," or "watch television"? Distracting yourself can be very effective—for a while. However, these strategies start to cause new and different problems if they are used to stop negative feelings altogether or to never pay attention to them. You can't completely turn off feelings without paying a high price. The feelings can be *put* away, but they don't completely *go* away. If we do not recognize and acknowledge our feelings directly, they will get expressed indirectly. Unexpressed feelings may result in our overreacting to minor difficulties, or our becoming emotionally numb (because when we turn off one feeling, the rest are affected as well), or diminishing intimacy in relationships (when we do not share our emotional lives, closeness suffers). Physical symptoms (headaches, muscle strain, ulcers, digestion problems) can also result. Even if avoiding feelings works most of the time, avoidance tends to fall apart just when feelings are at their worst and most overwhelming.

The solution we recommend is to allow yourself to feel lower levels of discomfort. Then you can learn to have some control over the more uncomfortable feelings. For example, trauma survivors often find that time alone means being flooded by painful feelings and images. If this happens, you may avoid being alone—for good reason. Feeling overwhelmed and unable to respond effectively to these negative feelings just repeats the feelings of going through the trauma. However, if you have self-comforting strategies that work for you, you are not helpless. You have an important tool. It is a gift to be able to enjoy time alone. This is how you can begin to reclaim that gift. Self-comforting is not about hiding or running away from negative feelings. It is about having choices. Self-comforting means you are taking care of yourself, even though you may not believe you deserve it. Not believing you deserve comfort and care is what many of the bad feelings are about. One key to using self-comfort as a coping strategy is to do it regardless of what you think or believe about yourself at the time. Taking care of yourself may not come easily—it may be easier for you to put energy into taking care of others—but if you are worn down, sick, exhausted, or overwhelmed from not having adequately cared for yourself, you will be less effective in caring for others.

Learning More about Your Relationship with Yourself

Are you aware of your own feelings—such as sadness, anger, happiness, satisfaction, frustration—either as they occur or some time later? Do you name these feelings for yourself or express them to others?

When do you become aware of your feelings? Do they have to be strong and powerful to get your attention?

Do you believe you have a good relationship with yourself?

How do you handle strong emotions?

Is how you feel and think about yourself constant? Or does it change, depending on whom you are with?

Do you ever experience feelings of shame and self-hatred? when?

What do you do to lessen those feelings?

What do you like about yourself?

Learning to Recognize, and Use, Dissociation

Many trauma survivors are familiar with dissociation. It is a coping skill used to manage overwhelming feelings. Some people with repeated experience of traumatic events, particularly during childhood, learn to dissociate early in life. Dissociation means emotional and mental escape when physical escape is not possible. For example, dissociation can mean not allowing the painful situation into conscious awareness. It might also mean blocking its emotional impact by mentally or emotionally compartmentalizing the trauma. This allows survivors to detach from the traumatic event, helping them avoid its total impact. If you dissociate, you may lose time—time that you cannot account for or time during which you are uncertain of your actions. When an event is too overwhelming, or the feelings become too painful to tolerate, it is natural and self-protective to dissociate.

❂ *As an adult, whenever Sally thought about the way that her brother abused her when they were children, she felt light-headed and dizzy and had difficulty focusing on the task or conversation at hand. Even as an adult, after the abuse had ended, she still felt afraid whenever her brother was around. She frequently had difficulty recalling all of the events and conversations that occurred during the times they were together because she tended to feel blank and numb most of the time he was around.*

You may have blocked off some aspects of your experience and remember others. You may still try to avoid emotions related to the traumatic events by dissociating, using drugs or alcohol or by escaping into your work. It is normal not to want to feel pain associated with traumatic experiences. In the long run, however, keeping feelings and memories beyond your conscious awareness can create difficulties in other parts of your life. If it is uncontrolled, dissociation interferes with your relationship with yourself. It gets in the way of enjoying time spent alone, comforting yourself, feeling good about yourself, or of tolerating strong feelings. Dissociation does not allow you the opportunity to develop alternatives. Even when you feel numb, blocked off parts of the trauma may limit your reactions and restrict your life choices. As mentioned earlier, shutting down negative feelings usually constricts positive feelings as well. Opening yourself to feel and face pain gradually can also open you to feeling joy in your life. Feeling anger can help generate energy for healing projects or changing unacceptable conditions. Your goal is to make dissociation a conscious choice.

Controlled or planned dissociation can be a resource. For example, when you are frightened, you may help reduce your fear if you are able to withdraw to an imagined protected place. This planned dissociation can help you gain some control over your fear. The chosen safe place may be in direct contrast to a place of darkness or aloneness that you visited during the trauma. Some people use planned dissociation during medical exams by focusing on written material around the room or conjuring up an image of something pleasant.

Controlled dissociation is not useful if you always use it to block a feeling and avoid feeling uncomfortable. There are other ways to regain comfort, but you will never give yourself a chance to find them if you only and always dissociate. In order to develop a stronger relationship with yourself, you have to be willing to tolerate feeling uncomfortable, even miserable at times. It may be frightening to imagine letting yourself experience your feelings. In fact, you may believe that doing so would disrupt your day-to-day life. You are probably right if you mean suddenly giving up all dissociation. But that is not what we mean. As we explain in Chapter 3, there are ways to think through a belief such as this and carefully plan a very low-risk way of beginning to test it.

If others are not aware of your use of dissociation, you may believe that you possess a secret, something that others must not discover. Your private knowledge may leave you feeling ashamed, isolated, or even crazy. If you experience struggles or feel stuck in this particular area, we recommend the book *Getting through the Day* by Nancy Napier, listed in Appendix A. A knowledgeable trauma therapist may also be a great help.

Do you believe you ever dissociate? If you think you do, try answering the following questions.

If you dissociate, are there particular times or situations when it occurs? when and where?

Can you ever control when and where you dissociate, or does it typically occur automatically?

If you dissociate, in what ways is it harmful? helpful? both?

Do you have a safe place inside yourself (for example, an image of an outdoor scene or other place, an image of yourself in a protective bubble, an image of yourself with someone who can protect you)?

STAYING SAFE OUT IN THE WORLD

Coping with negative feelings is only one way to take care of yourself. Protecting yourself out in the world with other people may also be an issue for you. Traumatic experiences may have left you feeling powerless over what happens in your life. Trauma can undermine your sense of competence or faith in your own judgment. You may feel defeated about protecting yourself, particularly in new situations. You may think, "Why bother trying?", "It doesn't matter what I do," or "Nothing I do makes a difference." If you believe these statements, you may find yourself on a dangerous street or you may subject yourself to emotional harm in unhealthy relationships. However, you have choices. You can choose to seek a safer route to get where you are going. You can take steps to protect yourself in the world and with other people. Have you ever considered this before? If not, think about it now.

What do you do to keep yourself feeling safe in the world?

Do you have a safe place outside yourself (for example, a room in your home, a friend's home, your therapist's office)?

When people believe that they cannot protect themselves, they may be less likely to take the necessary precautions for safety. If you believe that nothing you do would insure your safety, you would be unlikely to take steps to protect yourself. On the other hand, if you belief that you can increase your level of safety and minimize the risk of harm, you are likely to take the necessary steps to do so.

There are a number of ways you can take steps to be more protected from physical and emotional harm in the larger world. They are

- feeling emotional connection with other people
- handling feedback from others without feeling devastated
- anticipating consequences
- having appropriate interpersonal boundaries
- having mutual (give and take) relationships

Feeling Emotional Connection with Other People

Part of being human is needing an inner sense of emotional connection with others. This is our basic need for intimacy, and we will talk about this need in more detail in Chapter 8. Emotional connection is also one of the most effective ways of coping listed earlier in this chapter. Receiving support from others is a form of emotional connection. Following the trauma, you may find it difficult to hold onto a positive feeling of connection with supportive friends or therapists. The time when you most need support, understanding, and acceptance, is sometimes the hardest time to seek it out.

When you live through a trauma, you may feel all alone with your pain. It may feel like no one else can possibly understand what you're going through, perhaps even others who have shared a similar experience.

> ❧ *Andrea had several good friends with whom she enjoyed spending time. She often called them on the spur of the moment to get together. While on a business trip, she was mugged by a man who stole all of her jewelry and her briefcase, physically injuring her in the process. After this, she felt very fearful and seldom went out, other than to go to work. She stopped calling her friends and didn't respond to their numerous attempts to reach out to her. Andrea felt numb and unable to feel any of the warmth coming from her friends. She felt disconnected from all of her relationships, which left her feeling completely cut off.*

Andrea's terror overshadowed and crowded out her other feelings. Over time, she finally responded to one friend of hers who had experienced something similar years before. This felt like a safe initial connection with another person; Andrea believed that a friend who had been through it would be more likely to understand what she was going through without judging her or pressuring her to do things she wasn't ready to do. This difficult first step helped her begin to reconnect with the people who cared about her and whom she also cherished.

There is a range of ways to help hold onto a sense of connection with others. One way is to let those closest to you read Chapter 1 of this workbook to help them make sense of your reactions. You could also copy and give them Box 1.1, the "How Family and Close Friends of Trauma Survivors Can Help."

It can also be difficult to hold onto a connection with others when you are by yourself or when someone cherished is far away. Photographs of the person you are thinking about can help you remember vividly a treasured time together or just help you feel as though that person is not so far away. Rereading letters from that person or even listening to a tape recording of that person's voice, if you are able to plan for a separation by making a tape, can help retrieve a sense of connection or closeness. Looking at or using a gift received by that person can also be helpful. Remembering good times spent together or even writing a note to that person, whether or not the person will ever receive it, can also help you feel closer to that person in his or her absence.

What do you do to hold onto a sense of connection with other people, even when they're not with you?

What other ways might also be helpful?

Handling Feedback from Others without Being Devastated

Traumatic experiences can leave you feeling raw and especially sensitive to comments others make. You may feel that something is wrong with you because of your reactions.

> ❧ *Larry was shocked to learn that his coworker was killed in a car accident on her way home from work the night before. He remembered their last conversation vividly and could see a clear picture of her in his mind. Even a week later, it was impossible to do anything at work without thinking about her. He felt as though he was not returning to "business as usual" as quickly as his colleagues. When coworkers asked him about whether a certain project was finished, or whether he would be at a particular meeting, Larry felt angry and defensive. And when people commented that he looked tired or upset, he quickly went into his office, closed the door, and dissolved into tears.*

The week after the death, a therapist from the community came in to allow Larry and others to talk about how their coworker's death was affecting them. Through this process, Larry learned that the other people in his office were suffering too. He heard them describe feelings very similar to his, and he realized that their comments were not meant as judgments or attacks. He realized he had been misinterpreting nonverbal messages that were actually reflections of others' own unspoken grief.

In the absence of information, it is natural to make assumptions about what another person thinks, feels, or intends. But such assumptions can prevent you from asking questions to learn more about what is really going on. It is helpful to assume that there are all kinds of influences on the other person that you might not know about. This may help buffer hurt, rejection, or other feelings that otherwise leave you feeling disconnected from others.

How does feedback from others affect your self-esteem or mood? How do you handle feedback from others?

Do you now experience feedback differently than you did before your traumatic experience(s)?

How do you react when others give you feedback that is positive?

How do you react when others give you feedback that is negative?

If you have trouble dealing with others' feedback, you will find more to help you in Chapter 7, "Valuing Yourself and Others."

Anticipating Consequences

As noted earlier, one effective and protective coping skill is the ability to anticipate consequences. This skill requires thinking ahead about what might result from a particular action you take.

❀ *Megan tended to make plans at the last moment. She enjoyed having people over for impromptu gatherings, but her feelings were often hurt when peo-*

ple were unable to attend her functions. She saw their inability to attend as a personal rejection. Over time, she recognized that her spontaneous style was a drawback. If she really wanted people to come, she needed to plan ahead, so they could plan ahead. She learned to do that. Sometimes she went back to her old ways, but she tried to remember that not everyone shared her spontaneous style. Those that didn't come probably weren't rejecting her at all; they simply had other commitments.

And in another situation:

❧ *Rose often went out with friends on the weekend. As long as she was with a large group, she always had someone to talk to and enjoyed herself. Several times when she went to a bar with just one other friend, however, she felt self-conscious and drank more than usual. The morning after such an evening, she always ended up regretting some of her behaviors and choices, and she felt embarrassed.*

Some people have difficulty anticipating what the consequences of their actions will be. It can be tricky to think ahead to what might happen after you do or say something. Thinking ahead is a skill. If you don't know how to do it now, you can learn by paying attention to your past experiences. What happened when you made certain decisions or took certain actions in the past? You can also learn more by observing or asking other people. You can benefit from another perspective and another person's experience. The first step for both Megan and Rose is recognizing that something is not working; they keep getting hurt in certain types of situations. When they see this, they are in a position to figure out what they could do differently to get a different result.

If you don't feel comfortable discussing your problem or hurt feelings with another person, try this: When you notice that something isn't working, think through a past event but imagine it happening differently so that it turns out well. For example, Rose could imagine that things would have been different if two or three friends had come with her rather than just one. But what would have happened if she and the friend had gone to a movie rather than a bar? Where else could they have gone? What other things could they have done? Why limit her activities to a bar? What would have happened if she had said to the friend that she'd rather not drink. Perhaps they would have gone out and enjoyed each other's company in a setting in which alcohol is not served. As Rose imagined these various scenarios, some felt more comfortable than others. Some seemed more fun than others. Rose can use all this information to plan ahead for new and better ways of being with herself and friends.

Do you ever plan ahead? How?

Have you noticed a time when not anticipating a consequence has created a problem for you?

Has your ability to anticipate consequences been affected by your traumatic experience(s)? How?

Maintaining Interpersonal Boundaries

To have an interpersonal boundary is to know where you "end" and another person "begins." It is also to know that you have a right to allow and not allow others to enter your personal physical or emotional space. Maintaining appropriate interpersonal boundaries is an important self-protective coping skill. Figuring out comfortable and safe boundaries can be difficult for those who have experienced violations such as unwelcome touch or harassment and emotional abuse. Such survivors may feel a loss of power or control that can leave them vulnerable to future violations. A natural and protective response is to withdraw from others. Withdrawing in order to be safe can work; but in the longer term, it can interfere with meeting other basic needs such as trust and intimacy. It's a challenge to trust and be open after a severe boundary violation. Trust and openness include risks. Taking risks is much more difficult after you've been hurt, and yet risks can enrich life as well. Chapter 6 includes a more detailed discussion of boundaries.

Finding Mutual Relationships

Another self-protective coping skill is being able to enter into mutual give-and-take relationships. Individuals who have been in relationships marked by significant power differences and abuse may not know their rights and therefore may not know how to develop equal and mutually respectful relationships later in life. Abuse, degradation, and humiliation may seem normal, natural, or even deserved. Survivors of abuse may find themselves on one, the other, or both sides of abuse at different times or in different relationships.

> ❧ *Marjorie was in an abusive marriage for many years. Her husband put her down, blamed her for the way he treated her, and convinced her that, if she left him, no one else would want her. She finally confided in a friend that the abuse was getting worse—and, with a lot of support, she left him. Marjorie was then surprised to find she was drawn to other men who treated her poorly. She struggled to state her opinions and express her feelings in relationships. She had to constantly remind herself to speak up, because it felt most natural to her to fade into the background, agreeing with whatever the other person said.*

And in another example:

> ❧ *George appeared to his friends to be an effective and powerful man. As a child, and into his adulthood, his mother constantly cut him down and called his feelings and ideas "stupid" or "ridiculous." Despite his confident appearance, his mother's words always echoed in his mind. He felt emotionally isolated, even when surrounded by his wife, children, and friends. He created a protective shell to hide from his own overwhelming shame and sense of inadequacy, and he tried to control those closest to him. His family and friends felt unable to share any of their feelings or ideas with him. For those whom he most cherished, he unknowingly and unwittingly recreated the same humiliating environment in which he was raised. It was painful for George when he recognized this pattern, but he was then able to change his style and participate in more mutual, less controlling relationships.*

Do you have close relationships?

Do your relationships tend to feel comfortably equal (for example, you support each other, you make decisions together, you don't intimidate each other intentionally)?

What do you do to establish and maintain give and take in your relationships in a way that feels fair and equal?

How has the equality in your relationships been affected by your traumatic experience(s)?

A useful resource to learn more about how to recognize and state your rights in relationships is listed in the Appendix A, *Your Perfect Right*. This book distinguishes assertiveness from passivity and aggression, offering concrete suggestions for how to express your opinions and feelings effectively. We will also discuss more about rights, power, and control in Chapter 6. Chapter 8, "Feeling Close to Others," can help you look, in detail, at your relationships and how you might help them become more mutual.

TIME OUT TO RELAX

Learning to relax during the day is a comparatively easy technique to learn. It is an important technique as you do the hard work of healing. Another relaxation exercise is given in Box 2.1. You may use this or any of the self-care exercises whenever you feel stressed or overwhelmed. Remember, the sooner you notice yourself starting to feel stressed and use a relaxation method (your own or one from this book), the easier it is to become relaxed.

BOX 2.1   Relaxation Exercise

1. Begin by sitting comfortably in a chair with both feet on the floor and rest your hands on your knees or on the arms of the chair.

2. Now roll your eyes up as though you are looking above and behind your head. Then close your eyes as you keep them rolled up. (This takes your attention away from whatever you have been thinking about because it is not the usual position for your eyes.)

    Now you may do one or more of the following exercises. You may want to change any one of the images to make it more appropriate, personal, or soothing for you.

3. Imagine you are walking on a beach. You can feel the warm sand on your toes as you walk. You can see the waves spraying in the air. You can even hear the tumbling of the waves as you walk.

4. Now the sun is setting colorfully. You see a small boat coming towards the beach. As it touches the shore, someone you love steps out and comes to you.

5. You recognize that the person is a messenger for you. You are able to say anything you want to that person. You can ask for help or just be thankful that the person is there. You don't have to say anything. Perhaps the person brings a message to you. You can listen clearly to that message. Take your time with the messenger. You do not need to hurry.

6. When you are ready, you may leave your imaginary beach. You can open your eyes and speak. You feel that the time spent doing this exercise has been good for you.

7. You are now wide awake and ready to resume the activities of your day.

You may do this exercise as many times as you wish. You are in charge of the process.

This exercise is adapted from S. W. Osgood. *Abandon Yourself.* Washington, DC: National Institutes of Mental Health, 1978.

CHAPTER THREE

*T*HINKING THINGS THROUGH

THINKING: verb; to form or have in mind, to have as an opinion, to reflect on: ponder, to reason.

WE MUST DARE to think "unthinkable" thoughts. We must learn to explore all the options and possibilities that confront us in a complex and rapidly changing world. We must learn to welcome and not to fear the voices of dissent. We must dare to think about "unthinkable things" because when things become unthinkable, thinking stops and action becomes mindless.
—James William Fulbright, *The Arrogance of Power*

BREAK, BREAK, BREAK
  On thy cold gray stones, O Sea!
And I would that my tongue could utter
  The thoughts that arise in me.

—Tennyson, *The Beggar Maid*

MAKING SENSE OF YOUR POSTTRAUMA REACTIONS

In Chapter 1, we described the situations of Paul and Kirk who had similar serious car accidents. After Paul's accident, he felt afraid when driving, particularly when the conditions were similar to those in the accident—on the expressway, in the rain. But after several weeks, he no longer felt afraid except occasionally when he saw someone else driving erratically. Kirk, on the other hand, felt emotionally paralyzed following his accident. He felt too unsafe even to get behind the wheel. Several weeks after the accident, he still felt afraid when not at home most of the time. He felt fear crossing the street and in a crowded store where someone could bump him.

Why is there such a difference between their reactions?

Kirk and Paul experienced similar events differently because the accidents had different meanings for them. They reacted according to the lessons each drew from the accident—and they drew different lessons.

Person	Facts	Meaning	Reactions
Paul	Car accident	"You can't always count on people to drive safely."	Fearful, unsafe when driving in traffic, anxious
Kirk	Car accident	"I'm not safe anymore."	Generalized feeling of being unsafe in the world

Your reactions to trauma—your thoughts, feelings, and behaviors—are a result not only of the facts of the traumatic events, but also of what you think those facts mean. You can't change the facts of what happened, but the lesson you draw from the facts is probably not the only one possible. There is usually more than one meaning for any set of facts.

For Paul, the meaning of the accident applied only to driving, and primarily to driving in traffic. For Kirk, the accident meant he was always at risk, almost everywhere. These two individuals can each draw different meanings from similar events because traumatic events do not occur in a vacuum. They occur within the context of a whole life, including current and past experiences. A bad past experience can make a recent, similar event more troubling, whether or not you are aware of the similarity. In addition, if you are under a lot of stress or do not have support from other people, you may be more likely to experience a difficult event as traumatic. If we spoke with Kirk more extensively about the accident and other difficult times in his life, we would be likely to hear about other times that he felt unsafe. These old experiences may have left him more vulnerable to feeling unsafe in this new situation.

Healing from trauma often involves gaining a new perspective that allows you to see the facts differently. This chapter explains how to do that.

We start with a few basic distinctions that can usually be ignored in day-to-day life. Specifically, we look at how facts, meanings, and reactions are different but also connected. Later in this chapter, we will look at how trauma can disrupt the deeper beliefs you have about yourself and the world and what you can do about that disruption.

Sorting Out Facts from Reactions

Kirk's reaction to his car accident was to feel afraid most of the time. This is a common reaction to trauma. Although such fear sometimes goes away on its own, sometimes it doesn't. It didn't get better for Kirk. Part of the reason was that he didn't fully understand the relationship between the *facts* of a situation and his *reactions*. Kirk thought that feeling fear meant that he must at that moment actually be in danger. It is true that fear is an important signal to us that we might be unsafe. We need to pay attention when we feel fear. However, fear may not always accurately signal the risk in a current situation. It signals only a possibility of danger that must then be checked out. This can be especially true following traumatic events.

It is possible to feel fear and be quite safe, or to have no fear but actually be in great danger. Thinking you are unsafe, whether or not you actually are, can stir feelings of fear. Feelings of fear can call up thoughts of being unsafe. Sometimes these thoughts and feelings are so compelling that they appear to be like facts in the present; but thoughts and feelings often have to do with something in the past that you are remembering, or something in the future that you are imagining. If you imagine eating something that you enjoy, you may begin to feel hungry. If you remember someone yelling at you, you may feel tense or upset. Such feelings may then evoke even more thoughts of being unsafe. When Kirk felt fear, he would remember the accident and how much danger he had been in. Then he would begin to worry about harmful things in the future that might happen to him. Kirk felt and thought he was unsafe—but how unsafe was he, in fact? He thinks he knows, but he hasn't, in fact, checked to see how accurate his thoughts and feelings are in the present.

Thoughts and feelings give you important information about how to act and take care of yourself. It is especially important to pay attention to feelings of fear. However, it is also important to ask yourself if the fear is warning of present danger, or if it is based on the past or the future.

Sorting Out Facts from Meanings

Knowing all the facts in a situation helps us know how best to react. Unfortunately, we are often in situations in which we don't know all the facts. What was that noise in the kitchen? It's a fact that there was a noise, but what does it mean? Was it the cat getting into trouble? Or has someone broken into the house? It's hard to know how to react until we know what the sound means. Facts do not always carry obvious meanings. Even when we know the basic facts of a situation, and agree on them, we may not all agree on what they mean. This is because a single fact or set of facts can often mean more than one thing.

Is a bottle of water half full or half empty? The amount of water, eight ounces, is a physical fact that can be measured. This fact is independent of who we are, what we think or feel. But that same fact can *mean* different things to different people or even to the same person in different situations. If you are thirsty and believe there is nothing to drink, you can be delighted to find that there is still some water left in the bottle. If you believe there is a full bottle to share with friends, you will be disappointed to find it only half full. The meaning that the water bottle has for you depends on the whole situation. This includes what you bring to that situation, what you expect, what has happened to you in the past, and what you believe those past experiences have meant to you. *Meanings are not the same as facts.* There is no right or wrong meaning to the water bottle. There is not even necessarily one best meaning. It is possible to have many different meanings that all fit the same facts.

Kirk believed the meaning of his car accident was "I'm not safe anymore." He believed that this was the *only* meaning the accident could have. He knew he couldn't undo the fact of the accident and he thought meanings operated in the same way. They don't. A fact such as the amount of water in a bottle either is or is not eight ounces. It can't be two different amounts at the same time. Meanings, on the other hand, are the way we interpret what facts have to do with us, personally. It is very possible, and even probable, that something might mean two or more things at the same time and both can fit the same facts.

Let's look at another example. Cindy and Jack went through the same traumatic experience but it meant different things to each of them. Neither of them had any previous experience of trauma.

❈ *Cindy and Jack were walking downtown together when a man robbed them at gunpoint. The mugging left them shaken, but in different ways. Cindy had typically trusted her own judgment and felt that she could control events that affected her. Some time before the robbery, she had considered but then decided not to carry mace for self-protection. After the robbery, she thought a great deal about her decision. In her head, she went over each moment of the holdup. She focused on those moments in which she could have acted differently. She believed that if she had been better prepared, she might have controlled the outcome. The robbery disrupted her trust in herself and her usual feeling of being in control of what happened to her. These, however, were not the ways in which Jack was most affected. He had generally experienced his peers as trustworthy. He suffered tremendous upset because he had been robbed by a male approximately his own age. Previously he enjoyed relaxed and easy relationships with his friends and coworkers. Now, suddenly, he found himself feeling distrustful and suspicious of them.*

We can begin to make sense of their different reactions by looking at what the event meant to each of them. The meaning that each drew was based, not only on the mugging, but also on their separate histories and experiences. Jack had enjoyed good, trusting relationships with his peers. The robbery changed that for Jack because it meant his peers could no longer be trusted. Meanwhile, Cindy believed the following about herself, before the robbery:

"I make good decisions."
"My choices are sound."
"I am good at thinking things through."
"If I take these steps, everything will work out."

The first three thoughts reflected Cindy's overall sense of trust in herself. The fourth thought reflected Cindy's sense of having control over her life. She probably would admit that she didn't "always" make good decisions or that she couldn't "always" control how things worked out even though, to some extent, this is what she believed. But immediately following the assault, Cindy thought

"I always overlook things that really matter."

"Nothing I do seems to make a difference."

The change in Cindy's thoughts and feelings from before to after the mugging helps show where, why, and how the trauma has affected her. The mugging made Cindy question her earlier decision not to carry mace. This, in turn, made her question whether she could ever again trust herself to make good decisions. The risk of making any mistake seemed unbearably high after the experience of the robbery. She wasn't sure what to think anymore but the safest thing was to believe the opposite of what she had believed before; that is, she no longer trusted herself at all, she felt nothing she did made a difference. This is the lesson—the meaning—she drew from the trauma.

The trouble with this lesson is that it is a basic human need to be able to trust yourself and others. It is a basic need to have some sense of control over what happens to you. Your internal core is partly made up of a sense of trust, control, safety, intimacy, and self-esteem. This is why Cindy feels shaken to the core. *Traumatic experiences contradict our core beliefs about basic human needs.*

MAKING SENSE OF BELIEFS

Beliefs are meanings about ourselves, other people, and the world that we have come to trust and rely on very deeply. We develop these deep beliefs out of what has happened to us, what we've been told to believe, and from watching what happens around us. Children often believe what they are told: "Strangers are dangerous," "Listen to and respect grown-ups," "Don't burden people with your problems," "You're bad." If you witness violence in your home growing up, you may believe that caring people hurt each other, or that you never leave a relationship no matter how damaging it might be. On the other hand, your past experiences may have led you to believe that you are always safe, that you are in control of what happens to you, that others are always trustworthy, or that no matter what happens, things will work out okay in the end.

Because beliefs are meanings, they are based on evidence, past facts, and experience. They are the lessons we draw to help us know how best to act or react in the present. Once we've formed our core beliefs, we usually stop thinking much about them. They become a natural part of who we are and how we function. We tend to act on them automatically, as reflex. Cindy confidently believed, "I make good decisions." She confidently made the decision not to carry mace. The robbery shocked Cindy into considering that her deep belief might be wrong.

Beliefs can and do change. Most of the time they change gradually as the weight of our experiences shapes what we believe. The process is similar to the way a river gradually shifts its course as the surrounding terrain erodes. This process of belief change is called *accommodation*. It is possible to exert some control and influence over the process, and we will discuss strategies for doing this a bit later in this chapter. With trauma, however, basic beliefs can change quickly and dramatically, the way an earthquake can suddenly shift the course of a river. A belief may intensify, become absolute, reverse itself, or collapse altogether.

Immediately following the assault, Cindy felt that any trust in herself and control in her life were gone completely. She believed this as completely as she once believed that she always made good decisions. Were her new beliefs any more true and accurate than the old ones? Actually, no; the new beliefs have an "always" in them as well. As time went on Cindy was able to see that, in fact, she didn't *always* overlook things that mattered. Even though she was full of doubts about herself, felt out of control and helpless, she was able to make some small plans that turned out fine. She found ways to stay safe while checking out how much she really could trust herself. For example, she asked friends when she felt unsure about a decision and wanted other perspectives. Six months after the mugging, Cindy believed the following about herself:

"I make good decisions with the information I have; sometimes, though, it helps to get input from other people."

"I value what I know, but I can't know everything."

"Generally, I can make things work out the way I want them to. Sometimes, though, things over which I have no control happen. At those times, I do the best I can."

If Cindy continued to believe that she could *never* trust herself again, *never* make a difference, her life would shrink. For Cindy, one important step in beginning to heal was realizing that trust and control were not all-or-nothing. When she was able to consider the fuller range of possibilities for trusting and having control, she found ways to recover some sense of both trust and control.

The Trouble with All-or-Nothing Thinking

Survivors of trauma, like Cindy, often think in black-or-white, all-or-nothing terms. Overwhelmed with powerful feelings, they tend to feel completely safe or completely in danger, completely in control or completely out of control. This kind of thinking can occur as a reaction to trauma. When trauma shatters a basic belief it can seem best to believe the extreme opposite. It may feel most self-protective not to expect anything positive from yourself or others. If you thought you were safe and suddenly found yourself in a life-threatening situation, it may seem much safer always to assume high risk than to assume safety. You may then feel better prepared to protect or defend yourself.

> ❖ *When Hilda married, she had never before felt so cared for. She trusted her husband completely. It was a little over a year into their marriage when he first hit her. He was extremely remorseful, promising it would never happen again. Several months later, another violent incident occurred and more followed. Hilda couldn't believe the change in this man she had so loved and trusted. She had no way to make sense of his violent behavior except to think that, apparently, you could never really know or trust anybody. She began to view everyone with suspicion and distrust.*

After the abuse started, Hilda began to distrust everyone. She withdrew from others to protect herself from being hurt more. It was a way of coping. She had already been hurt. The stakes were high—as they usually are with trauma—and she felt totally unsafe trusting even a little bit. She began thinking of people as either totally trustworthy or totally untrustworthy. But no one is perfect and so she felt she could not trust anyone. However, trusting is a basic human need and not being able to do this causes its own pain and problems. Does Hilda really have to choose between the two basic needs of safety and trust? It seems that way at the start, but if you think about it more carefully, you can see that this is a false choice.

Hilda is assuming that it *is* possible to be totally and perfectly safe *if* she gives up trusting others—but this is not true. This is an imperfect and flawed world; there is no way to guarantee absolute or perfect safety for anybody, regardless of what they give up. However, this is not the same as saying that Hilda can never be safe. Safety is not absolute, but danger isn't absolute either. There are many ways to be safe, and many degrees of safety and risk. The same is true of trust.

Hilda doesn't have to choose between trust and safety if she can begin to think about the wide range of real possibilities between all and nothing. Trust can mean many different things and have many different degrees. After Hilda thought about it, she found she could expand from two categories (all or nothing) of trustworthiness to five.

1	2	3	4	5
Distrust completely	Trust for low-risk requests	Trust with medium-risk requests	Trust quite a lot	Trust completely

This translated in Hilda's day-to-day life and relationship with any particular person as follows:

1. *Distrust completely*. Avoids this person whenever possible, has minimal contact.

2. *Trust for low-risk requests*. May ask to borrow this person's tools when working on a house project.

3. *Trust with medium-risk requests*. May call this person for support after a bad day at work.

4. *Trusts quite a lot*. May ask this person to watch her daughter when she has a doctor's appointment.

5. *Trust completely*. Calls to talk to this person when feeling very upset about something.

These five (or potentially more) degrees of trust offer Hilda many more options. If everyone has to be either totally trustworthy or totally untrustworthy, she would end up with much less support and fewer choices in her life.

How Do You Think about Things?

Has your traumatic experience changed the way you think about some things? In which situations have you noticed this?

Are there situations in which you tend to use all-or-nothing thinking?

If so, how does this type of thinking protect you?

How does this type of thinking limit you?

What feelings, thoughts, or situations would be different if you had more than just two options?

As you continue through this workbook, try to remember that most things in life are not all or nothing, black or white. Real life not only has many shades of gray but also many other colors. Remember that every time you expand your thinking to consider a fuller range of possibilities, you also will have more options in how you live your life.

Accommodation: Understanding How Beliefs Change

As we have just discussed, the shock of even a single traumatic experience can suddenly change a core belief. Most of the time, beliefs change more slowly and gradually through the process called accommodation. When something happens, we automatically check the experience against our existing sense of ourselves, others, and the world. If the facts don't fit our beliefs enough of the time, those beliefs will gradually change to fit the facts. Our beliefs *accommodate* our experiences. The process is so automatic we usually aren't aware we are doing it.

Suppose you believe no one enjoys being with you. You would then not expect anyone to invite you out, say, on a ski trip. But what if someone did? What would you do with this new information? It does not fit your belief that people don't like you. At first, your belief would probably remain strong. You could find ways to interpret the new facts so that they fit with your old belief. You might tell yourself that you were only invited because they needed an extra person to help fill up the condo they were renting. Or they feel sorry for you because they know that no one else is likely to invite you anywhere. In other words, the invitation doesn't mean they, or anybody, really like you. If you kept getting invitations from these people, your belief that they dislike you might begin to change bit by bit. The belief would begin to *accommodate* the new facts. First, you might allow yourself to believe that perhaps one person enjoys your company, but that doesn't mean the others necessarily do. Over time, you might come to see that the belief that nobody likes you was based on outdated or incorrect information. Your new belief might be that you are likable and some people like you.

In order for the accommodation process to take place, there are two basic requirements:

1. You need to come into contact with facts that do not fit the belief.
2. You need to pay attention to that evidence while keeping an open mind.

These may sound like the same step, but they are different. Beliefs are based on past real experiences. Changes in beliefs come out of real experiences too. If I experience a robbery or a car accident, this is real-world evidence that contradicts my belief that I'm *always* safe. It's evidence I can't ignore. My belief may change to, "I am *never* safe outside my house." If I then never actually go outside my house, I will never come into contact with evidence that the belief could be wrong. Without evidence, accommmodation will never occur, even if the belief is inaccurate.

Actual experience, by itself, isn't always enough; we constantly filter or ignore experiences in our day-to-day lives. This is where the second requirement comes in: You must pay attention to evidence. This requires keeping an open mind. If you don't have an open mind, you will find it difficult to notice evidence when you see it. It is easy to dismiss, ignore, or explain away contradictory evidence automatically. This is natural, but not necessarily in your best interest. It is, of course, wise not to make big changes on the basis of a single experience. However, explaining away experiences as "exceptions" can happen so fast you may not notice what has actually happened.

Kirk's car accident made him believe he was not at all safe outside his house. Yet he did come and go safely, not just once or twice, but a number of times. He saw each time as a single exception that did not count. He didn't notice that over time, evidence was building that he was actually safer than he felt. If he had a more open mind on the question of his safety, he would pay more attention to the evidence over time. His beliefs about safety would have a chance to gradually accommodate the evidence more accurately and comfortably. He can speed the process if he knows how to keep an open mind and what to pay attention to. Later in this chapter, we will discuss certain circumstances that make beliefs even more difficult to challenge or change, even in the face of contradictory evidence.

Trauma and the Five Basic Needs

Trauma throws you for a loop because it changes your core beliefs about one or more of five basic human needs: safety, trust, control, self-esteem, and intimacy. We need some minimum amount of each of these things for ourselves and for those close to us. When we don't get enough of what we need, we can begin to experience distress.

Box 3.1 offers a basic description of what we mean by each of these needs. As we will see in Chapters 4 through 8, these are not the only meanings. Each need probably means something a bit different to every person. A key part of this workbook is to help you discover what these needs mean to you.

If you are experiencing troubling posttrauma reactions, it can probably be traced to a change in your thinking about one or more of these five needs. You may no longer feel safe or able to trust. You may feel out of control, worthless, or alone. You may have any or all of these reactions. If you do, your trauma experience has probably disrupted your beliefs about that need. What did that need mean to you before the trauma? How has it changed since the trauma? What lessons about that need did you draw from the trauma ? Are those lessons accurate? Are there other possible meanings to events in your current life? Perhaps you do not need to feel hopeless about regaining a sense of safety, trust, or intimacy.

BOX 3.1   Five Basic Needs Often Disrupted by Trauma

Safety for yourself: The need to feel that you are reasonably protected from harm inflicted by yourself, by others, or by the environment

Safety for others: The need to feel that people you value are reasonably protected from harm inflicted by yourself, others, or the environment

Trust in yourself: The need to rely on your own judgment

Trust in others: The need to rely on others

Control of yourself: The need to feel in charge of your own actions

Control with others: The need to have some influence or impact on others

Esteem for yourself: The need to value what you feel, think, and believe

Esteem for others: The need to value others

Intimacy with yourself :   The need to know and accept your own feelings and thoughts

Intimacy with others: The need to be known and accepted by others

Why Identify Your Basic Beliefs?

Your interactions with other people are automatically filtered through the screen of what you believe. Suppose you arrange to meet a friend who still has not arrived 20 minutes after the meeting time. If past experience has led you to believe that "I'm not important," you are likely to see her lateness as confirming your existing sense about yourself. You might think, "She doesn't value me," "I'm not important to her," "She must not really want to see me," and so on. If the experience means this then it may stir up feelings of low self-esteem, shame, sadness, self-loathing, or anger at the friend. You might storm away, feeling hurt and angry before she arrives because you believe her lateness means you are not important to her. All your negative beliefs about yourself and others will seem to be proven—but they aren't. You are actually jumping to a conclusion about the situation on the basis of insufficient evidence.

Your experience of the same situation would be much different if filtered through a belief that "I'm important," or "People enjoy my company." In this case, you might think that your friend's lateness means she has difficulty managing her time, or that something unexpected came up, or that she was caught in traffic. If you believe the friend values you, you would be more likely to wait until she arrives and then listen to her reasons for being late. This would certainly influence how you and she both felt and how the situation turned out.

When you learn to identify your beliefs, you come to know yourself, know who are are, and where you really stand. After trauma you may not know who you are anymore. Discovering what you now believe, after trauma, is a way to ground yourself again. It shows you choices you cannot see now but that are, in fact, there. As we will see in Chapter 6, knowing yourself in this way is a foundation for personal power. Coming to knowing yourself is not an easy task for anyone. It is especially difficult if you are afraid of what you might find out. This is why discovering your beliefs should be done slowly, carefully, and at your own pace. It should be done with a strong safety net of self-care activities. The first step in coming to both know yourself and care for yourself is to respect your fears and other feelings. Don't ignore them; listen to them. The rest of this workbook is designed to help you trace your trauma reactions to changed beliefs about your basic needs.

TRACKING REACTIONS TO THEIR SOURCE IN CHANGED BELIEFS

Most of us take our basic beliefs about trust, safety, control, self-esteem, and intimacy for granted, but traumatic events have a way of leading us to question such basic assumptions about the world. This is a key part of what makes trauma so uncomfortable. It can feel terribly disorienting and confusing.

> ❀ *Bruce was at the stadium when an earthquake struck. Thoughts flashed through his mind: Am I going to die? Will anyone be able to find me if the building collapses? Will I be able to escape if I get hurt? Although he had never worried much about these things before, he became preoccupied after the earthquake. He frequently had random thoughts about being injured in a variety of situations. He was often afraid. Only now did he realize that he had taken his safety for granted. He had believed he could control his safety but now he felt totally out of control. He felt as though safety itself was lost to him and he was now in great danger. Then he realized he must have been in danger all along, but only after the earthquake did it really sink in. His earlier sense of safety must have been an illusion; now that illusion was destroyed.*

Bruce isn't crazy to feel he has lost something. He has. He has lost his *belief* that he is safe. Has his *actual* level of safety changed after the earthquake? Probably not. He lives in an earthquake-prone area. There was risk before, and the risk will continue. What has changed is that he can no longer ignore the risk as he did before. Now that he sees risk, he believes he cannot be safe at all. He makes this connection automatically and isn't even aware of it. If he begins to pay attention to what he's feeling and thinking, he can become aware that he believes "If there is risk, I cannot be safe." Once he sees this, his fear makes more sense. He realizes that he believes "safety" can *only* mean zero risk. Therefore, any risk means he is not safe. Is this true? Is it possible to be safe in spite of some risk; and if so, what does that mean?

Risk is real. The need for safety is real. But neither is total. Neither is absolute. If Bruce keeps an open mind, he can begin to find out what it means to him to be "safe enough." He can do this by paying attention to all of the evidence, by continuing to ask questions, and finding safe ways to test both old beliefs and possible alternative meanings. He may find that he cannot feel safe unless he moves to a place that doesn't have earthquakes. However, this doesn't have to be the case. Many people feel they can be safe enough to have a full life despite being at some degree of risk.

When a traumatic event disrupts a basic belief, we see it first in our thoughts, feelings, and actions. By looking at those changed reactions, we can begin to discover the belief underneath that doesn't fit anymore.

How to Identify Your Basic Beliefs and Evaluate Them

The process of identifying and evaluating your basic beliefs has four steps:

1. pay attention to your thoughts and feelings in reaction to a situation
2. pay attention to the facts of the situation
3. identify the belief through which you screen the facts
4. evaluate the pros and cons of a particular belief

You can discover your beliefs by thinking through your reactions—your thoughts, feelings, behaviors—to a particular situation. In this workbook, we ask you to focus on recent situations that have presented problems for you. When you can sort out your reactions from the facts of the situation, the belief through which you see the situation becomes more visible. When it becomes visible, you can begin to evaluate its accuracy and usefulness. The process starts with paying attention to what you feel and think.

Pay Attention to Thoughts and Feelings.   Paying attention to what you are feeling and thinking is the easiest way to identify a belief shaken by trauma. A shaken belief will lead to changes in your thoughts, feelings, and actions. Suppose you experience a rush of thoughts such as "I better not answer my phone," "I can't imagine leaving my apartment," "That person behind me in line yesterday made me nervous when he talked to me." If you think these things, you are likely to feel anxious, fearful, or panicky. It might help you to stop and notice clearly that "I'm feeling very scared," or "I've been afraid a lot lately." What does it mean that you've been afraid a lot lately? What does this say about you? You may conclude, "I am not safe." This conclusion may *feel* like fact but it is an interpretation of one or more situations that may or may not be accurate. That is why it is useful to next sort out the facts of a situation. What do you know for sure and what are you assuming about it?

Pay Attention to the Facts or Evidence.   When you conclude that "I am not safe," it will feel true, like a fact. However, it is a "belief." A belief, after all, is something you believe to be true. Stay alert to the evidence. Does your belief match the current facts? What are the facts? Can you separate the facts from what you think they mean? What assumptions are coloring the way you interpret the facts? Facts include things that were said or done. Things that are observable. Facts do not include anything about meaning, motivation or intent, all of which are generally unspoken and open to interpretation.

Identify the Belief through Which You Screen the Facts. If you can see the difference between the facts of a situation and your reactions to those facts, you should be able to identify a belief that leads you to interpret the facts in a particular way. Beliefs are often so automatic that we do not take time to notice what they are. You can become aware of your beliefs, evaluate their accuracy, and examine their effects on your life. Understanding your beliefs and bringing them into consciousness in this way can be especially helpful for people who have experienced trauma.

Evaluate How Your Beliefs Help and Hinder You. Beliefs fit the facts of experience, but several different beliefs can fit the same set of facts. It is important to think through a belief in light of the factual evidence, but that should not be the only consideration. If you believe you are safe only inside your house, you will mostly stay inside your house. That probably *will* be safer than driving. How much safer, and at what cost? If you stay in your house, it may be harder to get other essential needs met, such as those for intimacy and support. You may become depressed if you stay inside most of the time. Do you feel you must give up one need in order to get another one met? Most beliefs have *both* advantages and disadvantages. If your beliefs have more advantages than disadvantages, that's good; but if they tend to hinder rather than help you, you almost certainly have other, better choices if only you can learn to see them.

Do you rate your beliefs as hindering you more than helping you? If so, we want you to entertain the possibility that other meanings might fit the facts. We ask you to try this in spite of how strongly you may hold your belief. Can you imagine doing this even if only as a mental exercise? Being able to imagine the possibility (not probability) of something different is what we mean by keeping an open mind. After trauma, it can be very easy to misread or misinterpret events in your current life. It can be easy to miss seeing all the facts, especially those that don't quite fit the belief.

When there are two interpretations that fit the facts equally well, you can choose the one that has the most advantages for you. You cannot always choose to change the facts of your life, but you do have some choice when it comes to how to interpret those facts. Each of the next five chapters asks you to evaluate your beliefs in this way and to consider what choices you might really have.

Pinpointing Problem Areas to Think Through Further

As you identify your key beliefs in each of the five need areas, you may find that many of your beliefs make good sense to you, match the evidence well, and have more advantages than disadvantages. This is good. You probably do not need to think more about these beliefs at this time in your life. Other beliefs, however, may not be working well for you. In each chapter, we will ask you to take stock and consider where you are in your work and how ready you are to continue. You may or may not feel ready to continue the process at that point. You should feel free to set this book aside while you take time for self-care and other aspects of your life.

A Note of Caution.   Testing beliefs can be enormously useful and liberating; it can also feel emotionally risky. Challenging old patterns of thinking can strip away some of what you've done to feel protected in your posttrauma world. If any belief or feeling is particularly frightening, consider that an important message. You may not be ready to think through those beliefs. You probably need further practice with self-care and self-comforting or additional support. If you still want to move ahead, don't try it alone. Find a qualified therapist with training in trauma to help guide you and keep you safe.

THINKING THROUGH A BELIEF

If and when you are ready to continue, we will ask you to think through a troublesome belief. We will ask you again to consider your thoughts and feelings and the evidence. Then we will ask you to take two further steps: (1) imagine possible alternative beliefs (or meanings) for the same set of facts and (2) plan how you can most safely collect evidence to check the accuracy of old and alternative beliefs.

The exercise, "Steps for Thinking Through a Belief" in each chapter, is designed to help you do this. These questions ask you to go over some of the same ground described earlier, but to think more deeply about it. Start by writing down a belief you suspect might be troublesome. What situations come to mind in connection with that belief? Pick one of those situations, then think through that situation and the belief using the following steps:

- Sort out the facts of what happened.
- Sort out the meaning the facts have for you.
- Identity the underlying belief.
- Evaluate the pros and cons of the belief.
- Imagine alternative meanings for the same facts.
- Evaluate the pros and cons of the alternative meanings.
- Consider how to check the accuracy of these beliefs.
- Put the process in perspective.

Sheila knew what it was like to be kept waiting by a friend. This had happened to her. By paying attention to her reactions in the situation, and asking what they meant, she had identified the belief that "I am not a worthwhile person." She decided to think this belief through more carefully. Box 3.2 (beginning next page) shows how Sheila did this and how she answered the "Steps for Thinking Through a Belief."

When Sheila had completed the exercise, she had a small piece of doubt about how she was seeing the situation. She was able to imagine alternative reasons for what happened. The more she thought about them, the more of a possibility they seemed. Maybe she was being unfair by jumping to conclusions. Soon after that, Sheila's friend called, apologized profusely and explained that she'd had car trouble out on the highway. She was hoping they could reschedule, as she was looking so forward to seeing Sheila.

This one episode will not magically give Sheila a new belief in herself. Beliefs change through accommodation, through repeated contact with evidence. But if Sheila pays attention to this evidence, it could be the beginning of an accommodation process that could lead her to feel a great deal better about herself. If she ignores this piece of evidence, then dismisses the next one, and the one after that, her belief in herself will probably not change.

BOX 3.2   Steps for Thinking Through a Belief: How Sheila Completed the Exercise

Sort Out the Facts of What Happened

Think of a particular situation or encounter that bothered you. Describe the "facts." What happened?

I had made arrangements to meet a friend for lunch at a specific time and place. I got there on time, but 20 minutes later, she still hadn't shown up or called.

Sort Out the Meaning the Facts Have for You

How did you interpret this situation? What did it mean to you? If you have trouble, think about your reactions first and ask why you reacted that way to those facts.

My friend does not care about me. She doesn't even care enough to call the restaurant and let me know what's going on.

Identify the Underlying Belief

What lessons did you draw about yourself? and about other people?

I'm not valued by other people. I'm not important. I'm not worth caring about. People take me for granted. Other people don't value me.

When did you start believing this about yourself? Was this incident the first time? If not, when and how do you remember first learning this?

It reminds me of when I was growing up; my mother always told me that I was no good, and that she didn't want me. She never seemed to cherish me or even enjoy being with me. She often left me alone while she went out with friends, even when I as really young.

Evaluate the Pros and Cons of the Belief

*How does believing this make you **feel** about yourself? What does it make you **think** about yourself?*

I feel sad and worthless, really low self-esteem in these kinds of situations. It feels like an awfully big reaction given the current situation, but I really feel unlovable, like "Who am I to expect anyone to ever really be there for me or care?" I think no one is likely to care for me or want me around. It makes me think I can't count on anyone.

How does believing this protect or help you?

I don't expect much from other people; as long as I don't hope, I protect myself from disappointment. But it honestly doesn't work very well. I tell myself, "See? I knew it." But inside, I still feel hurt and disappointed.

How does this assumption hold you back or get in your way?

I don't let myself get close to people; I'm so afraid that if someone gets to know me, they'll see the "real" me, and then know how unlovable I really am.

Imagine Alternative Meanings for the Same Facts

Look back at your description of what happened. Are there other ways to interpret what happened? What else could the situation mean? Is there an alternative meaning that would fit the facts of what happened? If so, what is it?

My friend was late. I guess there are a number of reasons that could happen. Sometimes when I'm late, it's because I've lost track of time, or misjudged how long it would take me to get somewhere. Sometimes something comes up at the last minute that I have to take care of before leaving. Occasionally I forget about an appointment, and I feel horrible when I put someone out because of my lack of organization.

Evaluate the Pros and Cons of the Alternative Meaning

What positive feelings do you have when you think about this alternative meaning?

It feels so much better to think that maybe it's not because of me that she's late. I feel better about my friend and a whole lot better about myself. I also feel hopeful that maybe my friends don't see me the same way my mother saw me.

What negative feelings do you have when you think about this alternative meaning?

I'm foolish to get my hopes up. It leaves me feeling vulnerable, and afraid of getting hurt again. I feel a little bit stronger when I have my emotional armor on.

Consider How to Check the Accuracy of These Beliefs

How could you test whether or not your belief is true?

I could ask my friend why she was late. I could even let her know that it's hard for me when she's late because it makes me begin to wonder if she reconsidered wanting to have lunch with me. Her response could give me a lot of useful information. I could

(continued)

BOX 3.2   Steps for Thinking Through a Belief (continued)

also try to remember experiences with other friends, and how much I've felt cared for or valued in other situations. I would also think about times I have felt that someone didn't care about me.

When you consider testing the accuracy of the belief, what are your fears? What is the worst that can happen?

If I questioned my friend, she could confirm my worst fears. I think that would devastate me. I'd feel like crawling into a hole and never coming out. I don't think I would hurt someone else. At worst, I might say things to her to make her feel guilty, like "How could you do this to me? You acted like my friend and then hurt me." And if I considered my other friendships, the worst thing that could happen would be that I would face evidence that I really am all alone in the world and no one cares about me. That would leave me feeling terrified.

What good things might happen if you test the truth of what you believe?

If I learn that others see me completely differently from how I fear they do, I might be able to gradually challenge my old beliefs. This would help me feel better about myself, and more trusting of and connected to my friends. I imagine it would feel wonderful to be freer, more honest, and less fearful in my close relationships.

Put the Process in Perspective

Will testing the belief matter 10 years from now? Would it help or hinder you for the future?

If I took the risk to speak with my friend and the whole thing blew up in my face, I'd probably feel ashamed and exposed whenever I thought about it for a very, very long time. I may also use it as evidence against myself for a long time to come. But 10 years? It probably wouldn't matter. And I may or may not even remember the whole incident, especially if it had a good outcome. If there were a good outcome, it could certainly have an impact in 10 years. Working on this issue could affect the direction of my relationship with others and myself from now on.

Adapted with permission from the work of Catherine Fine, MD.

WEIGHING THE EVIDENCE OF WHAT YOU BELIEVE

After you have thought through a belief and have imagined a better alternative, the accommodation process could begin to work all on its own. Sheila did pay attention to what happened. She noticed how her assumptions did not check out accurately. The exercise helped her pay more attention when similar situations occurred in the future. Because she was paying better attention over time, the evidence started to accumulate. The accumulated weight of evidence eventually began to change Sheila's belief about herself.

As we explained earlier in this chapter, there are two basic requirements for the accommodation process: You need to come into contact with facts that do not fit your belief; and you need to pay attention to that evidence while keeping an open mind. When these two requirements are met, the accommodation process can happen on its own. However, after trauma, one or both of these requirements may be missing from your life. It may feel much too risky and dangerous to be in situations that could test your belief. The strength of your feelings, and high degree of risk involved may also prevent you from attending to contradictory evidence even when it's there, or from keeping an open mind. These are valid and important concerns. Your safety comes first. *You should not try to collect evidence on a belief unless you feel you can do it safely enough.* This is why you need to *think ahead* and *plan* carefully before taking any actions.

Brainstorm Ideas for Collecting Evidence

Brainstorming is one approach for thinking up ways to collect evidence without taking big risks. Consider the task and then write down anything you think of that you could do, even if it seems unlikely, impractical, or silly. You may think that the only ways to collect evidence on a belief are high risk. This is usually not true. The high-risk ideas are often the ones you think of first. We do not want you to take any high risks. We want you to think up low-risk or manageable ideas.

Rank Ideas by Lowest Risk First

When you have written down a number of possible ways to collect evidence for the accuracy of a belief, the next step is to rank your ideas according to risk. The lowest risk idea goes first, followed by the next lowest risk idea. Once you have such a list, and it contains ideas that feel safe enough to you, then you can consider carrying out these evidence collection methods. Always start with the lowest risk method first. For example, the simple act of paying attention to yourself and others is a very low-risk way to begin collecting evidence on the accuracy of a belief. There are also others that build on paying attention to what is happening around you already.

1. Notice or observe events or actions and the people acting.
2. Watch other people's reactions to the event or action.
3. Notice when you yourself are already carrying out actions that produce evidence about your belief.
4. Ask friends questions about their reactions.
5. When it feels safe enough, take a small action with a safe friend and see how the friend reacts to you.

❧ *Carol's parents were extremely controlling and cruel. While growing up, Carol's parents never listened to her feelings or opinions, and always put her down. When she was upset or cried, she was severely punished, or sent to her room for hours at a time. She learned to conceal her feelings and act as if nothing bothered her.*

Carol believed that if she expressed her true feelings, she would be humiliated, abused, or abandoned. She saw the belief as true or false: She already had proof from her past that it could be true; what she hadn't considered was that the belief was not *always* true. If it was sometimes false, then it might make sense to learn as much as she could about when and under what conditions it might be false. Carol wrote down her existing belief:

I will be humiliated if I express my feelings to others.

Then she wrote down a possible alternative belief. She didn't actually believe this alternative but was willing to keep an open mind about it. This was her alternative belief:

It is safe to express my feelings to some people and in some situations.

The next task was to make a list of ways she could gather evidence for or against both beliefs. It was a challenge to come up with first steps that would have a small enough risk to feel manageable. It helped her to know she could start by simply paying closer attention to the evidence that already existed around her. No one else had to be involved or even know what she was doing. As long as she was just on the sidelines, there seemed no real risk of humiliation or judgment coming directly at her. But what kinds of evidence could she notice? She came up with four different things to simply observe before taking any kind of action that others might notice or react to. She listed first the one that seemed easiest and made her feel least anxious. Then she listed the others in an order of increasing anxiety. She was also able to think of a few small steps beyond those. When finished, her list of ways to test her belief went from least feared to most feared as follows:

Least Feared

Notice how other people express feelings.

Notice how people respond to other people's expressed feelings.

Notice what feelings I actually do express already ("I hate it when it rains all weekend").

Notice how people already respond when I express small degrees of feeling; for example, I could try this out with my boss, a coworker, a neighbor, or a store clerk.

Ask a trusted friend how she feels when I express a feeling.

Try to express a slightly stronger feeling (to test belief that my feelings are so different, wrong, or bad) with my closest friend or in another situation that feels safe to do so, to see what response I get.

Ask someone with whom I feel safe, how he or she feels when I express stronger feelings.

Most Feared

Carry Out Lowest Risk Ways to Collect Evidence

Carol's first four tasks were to pay attention to the evidence. For this to work, she had to be as objective as possible. This meant being able to sort out what she saw and observed (the facts) from what she thought or felt (her beliefs). The evidence would either support or not support her belief that expressing her feelings would evoke humiliation.

The first task on Carol's list seemed like it might be too easy to be of any help, so she was surprised to learn some things. She was usually so worried about expressing her own feelings that she didn't think much about what other people did. When was someone expressing a feeling, anyway? When weren't they? She began to notice how often people expressed feelings and that there were so many different ways they did it.

It was a little bit harder to pay attention to how people responded to other people's expressions of feeling. Doing the first step for a while made it a little bit easier in some ways. On the other hand, she found the second step harder in ways she didn't anticipate. For example, at first Carol ignored much of what she was seeing. When people reacted calmly, thoughtfully, or downright positively to another's expression of feelings, this behavior somehow didn't register with her. Sometimes she didn't notice at all; at other times she thought people were *pretending* to react positively but were harshly judging privately. In other words, she found herself discounting what she had seen. This is exactly what she was trying *not* to do and yet she still did it. She had not realized this would be difficult.

As Carol worked at each step, she began to notice something interesting. Each time she started doing a new, slightly riskier test, she felt some anxiety. But as she kept doing that test, and really paying attention to the evidence, she became less anxious about it. When she made her list, she thought her third, fourth, and especially fifth test were fairly frightening. But by the time she felt comfortable with doing the first two tests, the next ones were less difficult to imagine doing, and certainly less scary than they had looked initially. This was true even though she noticed that some people got upset when others expressed emotion—just as she had feared. However, as she kept paying attention, she also saw that not everybody reacted this way; and even when they did, they would usually get over it and it didn't seem to damage the relationships.

This is how the process of accommodation feels when it happens. Beliefs, thoughts, and feelings begin to change to fit the evidence of your senses and experiences. It takes time, and sometimes a conscious effort—and some beliefs are harder to change than others.

Record and Weigh the Evidence for or against the Belief

While you collect evidence for and against the belief, it is helpful to keep a record of what you notice and learn.

How Carol Completed the Exercise, Weighing the Evidence for and against the Belief.

A. *List a situation in which you noticed a belief you want to think through more thoroughly.* Last weekend I was planning to see a movie with a group of friends. Even though they asked what I wanted to see, my suggestions didn't seem to even get considered when everyone else decided they wanted to see something else. Once again, I felt like nothing I say or feel makes a difference.

What Evidence (Facts) Supports This Belief as Accurate?

1. My friends didn't seem to listen to my suggestion.
2. No one seemed to notice or care when I felt disappointed with the final decision.

What Evidence (Facts) Supports This Belief as Not Accurate?

1. My friends did ask me what I wanted to see. Maybe they were interested in my opinion, but didn't hear my suggestion in the midst of everyone else making their suggestions.
2. When I think about other times I go out with friends, it seems that they do care about what I want to do or how I feel about things. When I look back, it seems that my voice is often lost when I'm with a group of people. Maybe it's because I'm more soft-spoken than others, so people hear me better when there's only two or three of us.

After thinking through some of the evidence for and against your belief, you may find yourself more open to alternative beliefs or interpretations. How sure are you, at this point, that this belief (for Carol, that nothing she says, does, or feels makes a difference) is accurate? Mark how sure you are on the following scale. Use the second evaluation scale at some later date to check on changes in your beliefs in light of new evidence.

Date: _____

Accurate   Inaccurate

_____

100%   50%   0%

Date: _____

Accurate   Inaccurate

_____

100%   50%   0%

Troubleshooting When Beliefs Are Particularly Hard to Change

❀ *At 17, Linda was raped by someone she had just met. It was years before she told anyone what happened, and even then, she did not talk about it in much detail. At age 30, she still thought often about the assault, questioning what she could have done differently and blaming herself for not preventing it. Her belief that the rape was her fault prevented her from trusting herself with the men she met later. Whenever there was a man she liked, she fled as soon as he expressed an interest in getting emotionally or physically closer to her. She froze if a man asked her out or touched her, even in a friendly and nonsexual way. Over time, Linda grew increasingly frustrated with herself because she wanted to be able to develop a friendship or intimate relationship with a man.*

What prevented Linda from being able to change, given her awareness? There are four things that can make a belief particularly hard to change:

1. the feelings connected to the belief
2. how essential the belief seems to your safety
3. how much your past experiences have confirmed the belief
4. the age at which you developed the belief

It is helpful to recognize, in advance, when a particular belief has one of these qualities. Sometimes you can take extra steps to help yourself deal with it. Coming up against a particularly change-resistant belief can be frustrating, but knowing why it's hanging on can help. One of the problems Linda encountered was the power of emotions.

(1) *Feelings connected to beliefs can make change extremely difficult.* Beliefs learned through traumatic experience are usually attached to many feelings. Those feelings can make the difference between a willingness to test a belief and an unwillingness to even think about testing it. This is not about being stubborn or closed-minded. It's about self-protection. Once you learn what is painful and what is pleasurable, you are likely to seek out pleasure and avoid pain. The same goes for feelings. The feelings that warn or prevent you from testing alternative beliefs are your way of protecting yourself from repeating an experience that brought you much pain. A part of you wants to be very careful to not let the same thing happen again.

After Linda was raped, she believed that the rape was her fault. The following feelings arose from this belief.

Belief	Feelings
"The rape was my fault."	Low self-esteem, self-blame, self-loathing, self-doubt, fear, vulnerable, out of control, powerless

Linda's bad feelings about herself, and her fear, remained so powerful that she felt a continuing need to protect herself from being in that position again. Although she wanted closeness, her need for self-protection was even greater. She realized that developing a close relationship would require some risk on her part, as all relationships do. But the risk is unlikely to include the risk of rape. She began taking small steps to test out whether she could find ways of developing more closeness without feeling too unsafe or frightened. She learned that she could take actions to help her feel safer when getting to know someone. For example, when she dated someone she did not yet know well, she met him in a public place for relatively brief periods of time during the daytime and drove her own car. These strategies helped her feel less frightened and more confident.

Feelings are an important part of what can sustain your beliefs and actions. Emotions such as self-blame are a major obstacle to self-understanding, developing relationships with other people, and, ultimately, to change. If you pay attention, you are likely to notice things that you say to yourself without even thinking. These are automatic thoughts that reflect underlying beliefs and continue to influence how you feel and act. As Linda repeats the message to herself that "the rape was my fault" or "something is wrong with me," she makes it stronger. The feelings grow stronger too. Questioning the message helps but takes time. In the meantime, it helps to have more immediate ways to cope. Affirmations are one way to give yourself immediate help.

We talked about affirmations in the prologue. These can help to fight directly negative automatic thoughts and the feelings that go with them. An affirmation cannot by itself help Linda to trust men again, but they can help her deal with the powerful feelings of self-blame and low self-worth that overwhelm her when anyone starts to get close. In advance she prepared the following affirmation to help override the negative thoughts: "I'm not perfect but I still deserve love and respect."

Becoming aware of your negative automatic thoughts allows you to develop new statements to yourself that directly address the old beliefs. Affirmations are based on current information, life circumstances, and relationships rather than past abusive or unpredictable relationships or situations.

(2) *Beliefs are held most firmly when they seem essential to your safety, well-being, and existence.*

> ❀ *Lyle is afraid to disagree. As a child, he was hit when he disagreed with his parents. Now he believes that he must agree to be safe.*

Lyle's reason for believing that he must agree in order to be safe was real. But Lyle is no longer a child. Many other things have changed. His fear may still be strong but it's been a long time since Lyle checked how accurate that fear is now. Is the risk of testing it still the same as when he was a child? Recognizing that the answer is "no," makes the idea of testing the belief seem more possible. It also helps to realize that testing beliefs doesn't have to be an all-or-nothing process. There are many gradations of risk. Lyle's first experiment would probably *not* be disagreeing with his boss. The stakes might be too high, the power difference too great. Lyle could begin by trying small experiments in his life to test whether his belief is always, never, or sometimes true. For example, he might begin by disagreeing with a trusted friend about where to go out for dinner. When the friend suggests Chinese food, Lyle might be more in the mood for Italian. He could speak up with his friend and watch the results. Later, he could try something that felt a tiny bit riskier. Safety is the first, most important need to consider. Beliefs connected with safety are also among the hardest to change.

(3) *What you have learned from experience influences your beliefs.* The more your beliefs are confirmed, or agreed to by others, the stronger they become. Rita had very different family experiences from Lyle and her beliefs are also different. But they each probably feel equally strong about what they believe.

> ❁ *Rita was treated with respect when she offered her opinions at family meetings. Her parents listened carefully to what she had to say, and they considered her opinion when making certain decisions. She now believes it is good to express herself openly and she believes people will listen to her. She is now an open, vocal attorney.*

The strength of Rita's beliefs is based on her accumulated experience that the beliefs are accurate. If Rita's experience had led her to believe, "People don't want to hear about my feelings," or "People will reject or harm me if I express my feelings," she might not risk finding out how accurate those beliefs are. Without experiences to counter her beliefs, those beliefs will not change. This is why it is important to consider testing your beliefs in low-risk ways. Understand, however, that the more experiences you have had confirming the beliefs, the more experiences will probably be needed to change them.

Once you are aware of what your beliefs are, you are in a better position to test them. Testing beliefs about feelings can also begin with relatively low-risk experiments, for example, expressing a feeling in agreement with someone else. "Yeah, I feel angry when someone does that to me, too." If you try this, pay attention to whether the person just moves on with the conversation or whether he notices your feeling. Does he follow up on your experience? If he responds by asking more about what you felt, or how you handled the situation, he is expressing an interest and an openness, showing that he may be a safe person to talk to about your feelings.

(4) *The age at which you developed your beliefs influences their flexibility.* Generally, the younger you are when you develop a particular belief, the more difficult it is to change later; this is true whether or not the belief is connected to a trauma. The younger you are, the fewer prior experiences you will have had to counter the impact of a traumatic event. Furthermore, because of a child's developing nervous system, trauma has a greater physical impact on children. In the earlier example, Lyle's belief that safety required agreement was strong for three reasons: First, the belief concerned his essential safety. Second, the belief was confirmed by many family experiences. Third, the belief developed when he was a child. He could not know that his parents' response to him was not typical of the way others would respond.

To summarize, beliefs can be hard to change when the emotions attached to them are strong, when the risk for testing them feels very high, when you have had many experiences confirming they are true, and when you were very young when you started believing them.

Facilitating Change in Beliefs.   If you believe you are unsafe getting into a car, how can you change that? You begin by thinking through what you feel, think, and believe about safety. The following may help you think about each of the four difficulties in ways that can make change a little bit easier.

1. Emotions can be strong and should never be ignored, but they aren't always about here and now "facts." Self-comforting and self-care techniques can help lessen your emotional discomfort. It is okay to go slow and at your own emotional pace.

2. Don't take risks that feel too dangerous. Start with smaller risks. Chapter 4, on safety, talks more about levels and degrees of risk.

3. The more confirming experiences you have, the stronger the belief. However, be sure to ask yourself if the situation is still similar to those confirming experiences? What circumstances may have changed? How long has it been since you even tried to see if the belief is still accurate?

Understanding more about what makes beliefs hard to change can allow you to be more forgiving of yourself when change does not come as easily as you believe it should. Reminding yourself that you are experiencing normal, predictable posttrauma challenges can hopefully help you find patience to continue working toward feeling better.

We provide another relaxation exercise in Box 3.3. Having several options for ways to relax will help you find the approach that works best for you. We suggest that you first read through the script to familiarize yourself with it, as with the others we have presented. Once familiar with the steps, you may be able to do the relaxation exercise on your own. It may be easier, however, to read it onto a tape, or have someone whose voice or presence you find soothing, read it onto a tape for you. Take time out now to relax or find some other way to take care of or do something nice for yourself. Such an action can be relatively small and take only a few moments—for instance, imagining a peaceful scene—or a longer time, such as taking a hot bath or hike.

BOX 3.3   Time Out to Relax

Begin by making yourself as comfortable as is possible in your chair. Place your feet flat on the ground. Make sure that your arms are firmly supported either in your lap or on the arms of the chair. Make sure that your head is fully supported by your neck.

Now, I'd like you to relax your body as much as you can. Sit comfortably and just let go of any tension that you are feeling in your body. Take a deep breath (*breathe*), and let the tension flow out as you exhale (*let out the air*). Take another deep breath and just breathe out all your tension. One more deep breath (*breathe*) . . . and let it go.

Now let a warm feeling of relaxation flow into your body. Focus on your breathing. Become aware of your breath flowing in and out. Feel your chest rising and falling with each breath. Breathe naturally and smoothly. Feel the air flow into your body and leave it with each breath. Become aware of how your body feels as you sit comfortably in your chair. Experience the feeling of the ground under your feet.

Now feel the weight of your body where it touches the chair, and become aware of the support you feel from the back of your chair. Just become very aware of how your body feels right at this moment, with your breath gently flowing in and out.

(continued)

BOX 3.3   Time Out to Relax (continued)

Now, move your attention to your feet. Become aware of any tension that you may feel in your feet. Then just mentally try to relax that area. Let the tension flow out of your body. Feel your feet relaxed and warm. And then move your attention to your ankles. Experience the sensations in that part of your body. And as you become aware of any tension there, see if you can let that tension flow out of your body with your breath. Just mentally ask those muscles to relax. Feel that tension being replaced by a warm feeling of relaxation.

And then move your attention up your legs to your calves. Notice if there is any tension there. And if you feel any, see if you can just let it go. Gently will those muscles to relax. And become aware of a feeling of relaxation in that area.

Now move your awareness to your knees. And notice any sensations you may find there. If you become aware of any tension, just let it go. And do the same thing in the area of your thighs. Mentally check that area for tension. If tension is found there, just let it go . . . just breathe it out with each breath. And let a warm feeling of relaxation flow into your thigh area.

Now move your awareness up to your hips. And again, become aware of any sensation in that area. And let it go. If you find that tension remains in a particular area, don't worry about it. Just leave it and move on to the next area. So now focus your attention on your lower abdomen and buttocks. Try and relax those areas. Just let the tension flow out of your body. Do the same in your stomach area and be aware that you often hold a lot of tension there. You may find many sensations in your stomach. So just mentally tell those muscles to relax and see if you can feel the tension leaving your body.

Now bring your awareness to your lower back. Feel that area and experience the feelings there. If there is tightness in the muscles, try to relax them. Just try to let go of that tension. Do the same in your chest area. Be aware of any tightness. Just breathe it out *(breathe)*. Let it go. And let those feelings of tightness and tension be replaced by a warm feeling of relaxation. And then move your awareness to your upper back. Experience how it feels to lean against the chair. Feel that pressure against your back and see if there is any tension in that area. And again, if there is, just let it go.

Now move your attention to your shoulders. See if there is tightness there. See if your muscles are held tightly. Take a breath and let some of the tension flow out of your body with that breath. The shoulders are another spot where people tend to carry a lot of tension. So, if you continue to experience tightness there, don't worry about it. Just move on to the area of your neck. Feel that area. Become aware of any sensations there. Let go of any tension. Now bring your awareness to your chin. Mentally will those muscles to relax gently. And so, too, the muscles of your lips, your cheeks, your tongue. Just breathe all of that tension right out of your body.

Then check your eyes. See if there is any tightness in that area. Then check the muscles around your temples and your ears. Just feel the area in your forehead and let any of the tension you may find there go. Mentally examine the back of your head, right on up to the top of your head. See if you can become aware of any tension that you may be holding in your scalp. Then just let that tension be replaced by a warm wave of relaxation.

And now, become aware of how your entire body feels. See if you can become aware of the very warm, relaxed feeling beginning in your toes and reaching right to the top of your head. Again, experience the weight of your body firmly supported by your chair. Experience how your feet feel firmly touching the ground, gently supported by the earth. Feel your head, securely supported by your neck. Become aware of any areas of tension remaining in your body. Just acknowledge them and don't worry about them. Experience the warm, relaxed feeling throughout your body. Feel a comfortable, warm heaviness as you sit securely supported in your chair.

Now I would like you to return your attention to your breathing. While you remain as relaxed as possible, once again become aware of your breath entering and leaving your body. Become aware of the gentle rise and fall of your chest with each breath. Become aware of the air entering through your nostrils or mouth and the feeling of that warm air as it leaves your body. Just continue to breath naturally and gently. Become aware of the gentle rhythm of your breath, flowing in and then flowing out of your body.

Now, as you continue breathing and remain relaxed, I would like you to think of a word or a sound or a phrase that has a peaceful meaning to you. It could be a word such as "peace" or "love" or "God." You might also choose a neutral word such as "one." Take a minute to think of a word or phrase that has a calming and peaceful feeling to you.

(PAUSE.)

Now that you have selected your word or phrase, begin trying to silently repeat your word or phrase as you exhale. As you breathe in, feel the air enter your body. As you

(continued)

BOX 3.3   Time Out to Relax (continued)

breathe out, silently repeat your word. Continue doing this for a few minutes. As you find your mind wandering, simply bring your attention back to your breathing and back to your word. It is inevitable that distracting thoughts will arise. In fact, it is very common to find that you mind has wandered for several minutes. But don't let that bother you. Just remember to bring your attention, once again, back to your breathing. Remember not to judge your performance. This exercise does not have to be done perfectly. It does not have to be done expertly or skillfully. All you have to do is do it to the best of your ability. It will still be effective. So just continue breathing naturally and gently. Continue repeating your word or phrase as you exhale. Now practice this exercise in silence for several minutes.

(PAUSE.)

When you feel ready, gently open your eyes. You will feel calm and relaxed. You are now ready to continue your day, begin or continue work in your workbook, or turn your attention to a new activity.

Developed by Carol Reinert, MA, LCDP, and Dena Rosenbloom, PhD. Used with permission.

CHAPTER FOUR

FEELING SAFE; BEING SAFE

YOUR NEED FOR SAFETY: The need to feel that you are reasonably protected from harm inflicted by yourself, by others, or by the environment; the need to feel that people you value are reasonably protected from harm inflicted by yourself, others, or the environment.

OUT OF THIS NETTLE, danger, we pluck this flower, safety.

—Shakespeare, *Henry IV*

HOW SAFETY CAN BE AN ISSUE AFTER TRAUMA

Everyone needs to feel safe, secure, and relatively invulnerable to harm. Everyone also needs to feel that loved ones are relatively safe and protected. Traumatic experiences may rob you of your sense of safety and security in the world. Some survivors feel this lack only briefly, in situations that remind them of the trauma. Others feel completely unsafe most of the time. If you grew up in an unsafe environment—whether in a violent home or neighborhood or in a region ravaged by war—your sense of safety and security may be very fragile. If you experience traumatic events later in your life, you may lose completely your sense of safety for a period of time. Feelings of being in danger are powerful and uncomfortable. They may feel confusing or make you feel crazy. But they do make sense in the context of trauma.

❀ *Eleanor was in a serious traffic accident. Her new car was demolished, but she was not hurt. However, she decided to go by ambulance to the hospital "just to be checked out." She had a few bumps and bruises and was sent home by taxicab. Images of the accident haunted her dreams and thoughts six months later. She quit her job, taking a significant pay cut, in order to avoid a 20-mile commute, driving only when necessary. She does not feel*

safe as either a driver or passenger in an automobile. When she rides with
another driver, she becomes hypervigilant and overreactive. She is now a
"white knuckle" rider.

Although Eleanor did not suffer serious physical injury in the car accident, she easily could have died. Now, every time she gets into a car, she feels
she is risking death. There is a hard truth to this that most people prefer to
avoid: We are always, more or less, at risk for death. The more actively we
live, the more at risk we place ourselves. In truth, living cannot be totally risk
free and no matter how careful we are, we will all eventually die. Does being
safe mean the same thing as not being at risk? If Eleanor believes this, it
makes sense that she also feels unsafe all the time. But many people are able
to feel safe despite knowledge of some risk. What, then, can it mean to be
safe?

Trauma Survivors Speak about Safety

• Safety is self-knowledge, self-understanding, self-acceptance, and self-
responsibility. I develop it by first knowing myself and then applying this
knowledge to accept myself and my life history. Only after doing so am I
able to accept responsibility for myself. Doing so secured my safety.

• To write about safety is to write about struggle. Most people think of
safety as the end result of following rules or the correct use of equipment,
such as looking both ways before crossing the street, fastening your seat belt
or taking precautions on the job. If we remember to follow the rules or use
the equipment properly, chances are we will be safe.

But this safety is all external, it hinges on situations encountered in a
physical world. The safety that is most difficult to attain and sustain is an inner sense of safety. This is the struggle. It is never-ending. It is daily. It is
often hourly. . . . Safety can be an all-consuming issue or it can become a
complete nonissue. As long as the struggle continues, the issue continues
since the struggle itself is an act of will, the desire to make it one more hour,
one more day or one more week. Safety is a simple word that many people
take for granted. For survivors of abuse, life on the streets, riots, war, natural
disaster, or some other trauma, talk about safety is of utmost importance.

• If some part of you keeps a constant vigil, perhaps you need someone
to help you with your heavy load. If you have already found a safe place, you

may want to make it bigger, more permanent and positive. You can look for ways to take safety with you . . . a special rock or keepsake, hidden in your pocket, always there to touch; maybe a stuffed animal, waiting faithfully in a gym bag, just in case you need it. Write down the special places, times of the day or night, people, things, or activities that help you feel safe—working out, sitting in the rocking chair, painting, listening to music, walking the dog, visiting your best friend. See which of them helps you feel safer anytime, anyplace, or only in certain situations.

Is Safety a Problem for You?

Take a moment now to think about your own safety and your sense of the safety of people you love. How do you answer the following questions?

I *never* worry about my physical safety	___ yes	___ no
I worry *a lot* about my own physical safety	___ yes	___ no
My feelings or impulses sometimes frighten me	___ yes	___ no
I worry *a lot* about the safety of the people I care about	___ yes	___ no

If you answered "yes" to any of these questions, you may have concerns with safety. If you *never* worry about your safety, that can be an even more dangerous problem than worrying a lot.

WHAT CAN SAFETY MEAN?

Safety is not absolute. There are degrees of safety just as there are degrees of danger. The meaning of "safe" can change from one person or situation to another. Depending on the specific danger, there is a range of ways that a person can feel safe. To some people, feeling safe means being secure and secured, inside a well-defended, impenetrable fortress. For others, feeling safe could mean having a good escape route—the ability to run away. Both can work to help keep you free from harm. For some, feeling safe means having a trustworthy guardian or defender, whereas for others it means relying mainly on oneself. Feeling safe can also mean knowing how to avoid danger through taking care and exercising caution. Or it can mean having the right kind of protection for approaching danger safely.

What feels safe or unsafe for you will be connected to what you believe about the other needs that trauma can affect—self-esteem, trust, intimacy, and control. These other needs will probably also come up as you complete the exercises in this chapter. When you have worked on other chapters, you can revisit this one and see if your ideas about safety have changed.

For most people, being safe means not feeling afraid. For most of us, the absence of fear means absence of danger; feeling fear signals a heightened danger. When fear works this way, it is very useful. It alerts us to danger so we can take steps to protect ourselves. Trauma, however, can disrupt the usual connection between *feeling* safe and *being* safe in two ways: You may feel afraid without being in any great physical danger, or you may feel physically safe in a truly hazardous situation. Tina experienced the latter.

❧ *Tina had been hurt in various ways while growing up, and she needed to believe she had been, and still was, safe and able to protect herself from harm. In reality, however, she placed herself at great physical risk. She sometimes walked alone late at night in dangerous neighborhoods. She blocked out any awareness of the danger. When she was eventually mugged, she wrote it off as bad luck, attributing it to "being in the wrong place at the wrong time." She ignored any real danger in her behavior or the situation. It was easier not to think too carefully about the mugging than to accept the possibility of real danger in her environment now and as it had been when she was a child.*

Tina seems to be having a completely different reaction to trauma from Eleanor, the "white knuckle car rider" described earlier. Although Tina, at times, feels safer than she really is, Eleanor at times feels more afraid than the real risk warrants. Both think that safety is an all-or-nothing state. Eleanor always feels unsafe in a car. Tina believes she is always safe, even alone at night in a dangerous neighborhood.

But being safe or unsafe is not an all-or-nothing state, nor is it an always-or-never condition. Feeling safe means safe here and now, in the present. As life circumstances change, so too can conditions of safety. However, as conditions change *you* also can change, taking steps to keep yourself safe. This is why we have listed being flexible as the first guideline for coping with stress (see Chapter 2). Being flexible can work.

After trauma, feelings of fear may not change even when the situation becomes safer. This is what happened to Eleanor. She was in great danger during her car accident. These strong feelings continued into new and different situations. People who suffered trauma as children also can continue to feel fear despite changed circumstances.

✿ *Whenever Peter thought about his uncle abusing him as a child, he shook with fear. It made him feel extremely small and helpless. As a child, he had been small and vulnerable. His uncle had been much bigger. But time and circumstances had changed. He was, in fact, no longer so small. It helped him just to realize this and remind himself that he was an adult now and no longer small.*

The saying "time heals all wounds" is true for a number of situations. Sometimes, however, time by itself is not enough. Some of the exercises later in this chapter are designed to help you check whether your feelings of fear or safety match the level of danger in a here-and-now situation.

DIMENSIONS OF SAFETY

There are three situations in which it is important to think about safety and becoming safer. They are: being safe with yourself, being safe with other people, and being safe out in the world. Think about each one right now.

Being Safe with Yourself

How safe do you feel with yourself? Negative emotions from inside can feel extremely dangerous. As we mentioned in Chapter 2, these emotions can include the urge to physically harm yourself. If you feel an impulse to do this, or if you feel threatened by out-of-control feelings, you can act to make yourself safer. Many strategies for protecting yourself from harmful feelings or impulses have been described in Chapter 2 and in the tips for self-care section of the prologue. Self-comfort, self-care, and coping are all aspects of the same thing—they all help you feel and be safe with yourself. When you feel endangered by emotions within you, you make yourself safe by using strategies that work for you. When you understand what things comfort you and make you feel safer, you can use them in many different situations.

❧ *When Esther was feeling especially sad and despairing, it was difficult for her to get through the workday. She withdrew from friends, became increasingly isolated, hopeless, and felt utterly unlovable. What would have been most helpful for her at these times felt impossible; that is, to reach out to people who might care about her. When she felt this way, she would make herself think of something nice she could do for herself. Maybe she could take out dinner from a restaurant she liked, walk to a favorite place, or soak in a hot tub. When she did these things to comfort herself, it became easier to give a friend a call and reconnect.*

Being Safe with Other People

It is also important to be safe in your interactions with other people. The people you knew before the trauma may be affected by what you have been through. You may feel misunderstood, even by family or old friends, or you may feel unsafe with people with whom you once felt safe. You may find yourself deepening friendships with people who were once only acquaintances, as your feelings and needs change in relationships. You may also find yourself needing new friends. However, this can feel like a difficult time to risk making new friends. For this reason, it can help to find a therapist who understands trauma or to find a support group of other trauma survivors. You need to feel safe in at least one relationship while you heal and find ways to reconnect with family and old friends. You need to feel safe, but you also need to respect your feelings of fear. How accurate are your feelings of safety? How accurate are your feelings of fear? You can begin to reality-check your feelings of safety and fear with other people. We talk later in this chapter about how to do that.

Being Safe out in the World

It is important to be safe as you move around in the physical world. How accurate are your feelings when it comes to safety in your environment? If you feel either fearless, or heavy with fear, the feelings may not be accurate. When in doubt, choose the safer course. Understanding that feelings of fear may be inaccurate will not by itself change the way you feel, but it is a first step. In the meantime, it can help you be safer.

Other Aspects of Safety

Even if you are not in immediate danger, witnessing or hearing about a traumatic event can erode your sense of personal safety. This indirect exposure evokes feelings and images of the events, whether you are a bystander, rescue worker, or compassionate listener. Even the examples in this workbook, which help illustrate the concepts we wish to convey, may be upsetting. If you already have a disrupted or fragile sense of safety, additional exposure to danger may reinforce unsafe feelings, as happened to Matt:

❀ *While Matt was growing up, his father was explosive and violent. Matt often felt unsafe during the years he lived with his parents. As an adult, he chose to be a firefighter so that he could protect others from harm. Initially, he felt a boost every time he intervened in a violent situation, responded to a medical emergency, or rescued someone from a burning building. Eventually, however, his cumulative exposure to traumatic situations led to a feeling of personal vulnerability.*

A runner who injures his ankle can heal and run again, but the ankle may always be vulnerable to future sprains. Knowing that the ankle may be weak helps the runner to take better care of it and avoid further injury. An awareness of vulnerability can actually increase safety and self-protection and decrease the likelihood of additional injury. Ignoring injury, whether psychological or physical, can lead to problems.

❀ *Suzy came into therapy after she had been a passenger in a minor automobile accident. Although no one was seriously hurt, she had a traumatic reaction to the accident. She was intensely afraid of future accidents and developed a general fear that something terrible was about to happen to her. She became confused and frightened by her tremendous reaction to the relatively minor accident. She was from Bosnia and had lived in a war-torn environment prior to her emigration. She had never discussed her war experiences and had hoped to leave them behind when she left home. But Suzy's car accident brought to the surface all of her unprocessed memories and all the accompanying unresolved feelings from her childhood experiences. These included a history of severe family abuse. She had witnessed and tried to break up violence between her parents. Once she understood the roots of that reaction in her history, she better understood her present internal turmoil and reactions.*

In the following exercises, you will have the opportunity to examine your own beliefs about safety more closely. We encourage you to think of what enhances or diminishes your personal sense of safety.

As you answer the questions we ask about safety, you may feel many emotions. We encourage you to work at your own pace. Whenever you wish, stop and take a break, put the workbook aside. Feel free to skip certain questions, stop to write in a journal about what thoughts and feelings come up as you complete the questions, or take time to nurture yourself with a self-care activity (meditation, relaxation, taking a walk, calling a friend, listening to music, etc.). Healing consists of alternating states of readiness for moving ahead, times for digesting what has been done, and shifting focus temporarily when necessary. There is no right or wrong way to heal. What is important is that you do it *your* way, respecting your own personal pace, feelings, and needs.

WHAT DOES SAFETY MEAN TO YOU?

There are many different ways to define "safety" and many shades of gray for each definition. Plus, feeling (emotionally) safe and being (physically) safe are not always the same thing. Think about the different aspects of safety described so far in this chapter, then try to answer the following questions:

What does being "safe" mean to you?

With whom do you feel safest?

What things make this person safe?

A safe place is one in which you can feel comfortable, without fear. The smells, sounds, sights, physical sensations, tastes, and location of the place bring you a feeling of security. Do you have a favorite place in the real world where you feel safe and relaxed? Where is your safe place?

If you don't have a real, physical safe place, can you imagine a place where you would be most safe? If you have a real safe place, can you imagine how it might be even safer? In the box below, create your real or imagined safest place. You can make a collage of pictures and use photographs. You can write down words that stand for safety or you can draw a picture of your safe place. This place could be surrounded by sprawling fields, valleys or by barbed wire, high fences, a moat, rocks, or any other protective device. You may design it any way you wish. Imagine and create what brings you a sense of security. How would you design a safe place? (Use a different, larger piece of paper if you wish.)

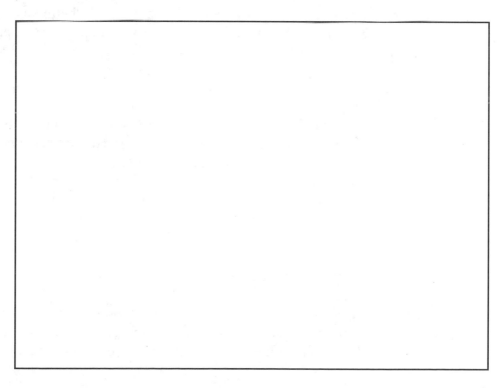

Look at your design. Is there only one thing that makes it safe or are there many things that together make the place safe? List the various qualities or conditions that make a place "safe" for you:

We think it is important for you to have a sense of safety before you do any work that looks at your lack of safety or beliefs about being unsafe. Some of the questions later in this chapter ask you to do that. When you come to answer them, it can help to go to your favorite, real safe place. If that is not possible, you could imagine yourself in the safe place you have just designed. It's easier to reach an imagined safe place when you are relaxed. If you have difficulty going there, try doing all or part of one of the relaxation exercises in this book. You can also make it easier to reach if you practice. Imagine your safe place often, complete with its sounds, smells, and scenery. The more you practice, the more accessible this place will be to you when the need arises. Whether in your mind or in reality, we hope your safe place is in easy reach.

SORTING OUT FACTS ABOUT SAFETY FROM YOUR REACTIONS

In the real world, there is no absolute and perfect safety. The facts are that safety coexists with danger. Most of us live everyday with some mixture of security and risk. Very rarely is anyone completely safe, or completely in danger. How well do your feelings, thoughts, and behaviors match the present facts of safety and danger in the world around you? After trauma, your reactions may or may not be an accurate guide to safety or risk in present situations. The exercises in this section are designed to help you sort your reactions from present facts and then see if they match. This is important information for you to have if you are to keep yourself safe.

How do you feel right now? Do you feel 100 percent safe? In other words, do you feel at zero risk of any harm? Or do you feel 100 percent unsafe with zero safety and a certainty of being harmed? On the following scale, circle the number that describes how safe you feel right now:

Totally safe,							Zero safety,
zero danger	1	2	3	4	5	6	in total danger

Did you circle 1 or 6? If so, you probably see danger and safety in all-or-nothing terms. It is likely that these extreme feelings do not match the facts of your present situation. Knowing this will probably not change how you feel, but it is important for you to know that your feelings may not match current circumstances.

Did you circle a number between 1 and 6? If so, you have some ability to see that safety is not all or nothing. This is good. Most of the exercises that follow in this workbook ask you to consider a range of responses between all and nothing.

Regardless of how you feel right now, you will probably feel a different mix of safety and danger in a different situation. In Exercise 4.1, we want you to think about whether your emotional reactions are different in different situations. Do you feel completely safe or completely unsafe in every situation? Or do you feel varying mixtures of safety and fear depending on the situation?

How Safe Do You Feel?

Exercise 4.1, "Rating How Safe You Feel" (see next page), lists a number of common everyday situations. Focus on the way you have recently felt in these different situations. *Do not think of any traumatic situation for this exercise.* Can you remember a specific recent incident or occasion? When was the last time you were in this kind of situation? How secure and relaxed (safe) did you feel? Or how tense and afraid (unsafe) did you feel? Complete Exercise 4.1 now, and then continue reading.

Where did you mark your answers on Exercise 4.1? If your responses were not all 1s or 6s, and varied from line to line, then you were able to identify differing degrees of safety in different situations. It is normal for feelings of safety and fear to vary depending on the situation.

Look now at those situations you marked as most safe. What is it about these situations that helped you feel even a little bit safer? Perhaps it is having a trusted family member or friend with you? Perhaps it is being in famil-

EXERCISE 4.1   Rating How Safe You Feel

Circle the number for how safe or unsafe you *feel* in each of the following situations. Think of recent common situations from your day-to-day life. *Do not use a traumatic situation for this or any exercise in this book.* Focus on your emotional reactions, not on your rational thoughts about the risk. If you think of other nontrauma situations in which you feel particularly safe or unsafe, list those in the blank spaces at the bottom of the exercise and then rate them.

Circle

1. Extremely safe	4. Somewhat unsafe
2. Moderately safe	5. Moderately unsafe
3. Somewhat safe	6. Extremely unsafe

How safe do I feel	Extremely safe					Extremely unsafe
at home with friends or family	1	2	3	4	5	6
at home alone	1	2	3	4	5	6
driving my own car	1	2	3	4	5	6
as a passenger in someone else's car	1	2	3	4	5	6
at work or school	1	2	3	4	5	6
on an airplane, boat, or train	1	2	3	4	5	6
with family outside my home	1	2	3	4	5	6
with friends outside my home	1	2	3	4	5	6
around strangers outside my home	1	2	3	4	5	6
alone outside my home	1	2	3	4	5	6
_____	1	2	3	4	5	6
_____	1	2	3	4	5	6
_____	1	2	3	4	5	6

iar surroundings? Perhaps it is being alone? If you can identify what is already working to help you feel safer, you can later use it as a strategy for feeling safer in other kinds of situations.

Take Time Out for Self-Care

Take some time to notice how you feel right now. Which questions stirred up uneasy feelings, and which were easier to answer? Noticing your feelings, without trying to erase or ignore them completely, is an important part of your healing. Noticing your feelings lets you know when to take care of yourself before the emotions begin to overwhelm you. Do you need to set this work aside for awhile? Do you need to take care of yourself right now? Do what you need to do to care for yourself. When you feel you are ready, continue.

How Safe Do You Think You Are?

Earlier in this chapter we explained that feelings of fear or safety are important signals, but they do not always reflect present reality. The next exercise helps you begin to sort this out. In Exercise 4.2 (see next page), we ask you to think about the same situations you just did, but this time try to put your feelings aside. Try to ignore, for the moment how safe or afraid you "feel" and instead consider objectively how safe or unsafe you think you really are in each situation. In other words, try to evaluate how likely or unlikely you are to come to physical or emotional harm in each situation.

Let's compare how you rated "feeling safe" and "thinking safe." Look at Exercise 4.1. Write down here the situations in which you *feel* safest:

_____

_____

Look now at Exercise 4.2. Write down here the situations where you objectively *think* you are safest:

_____

_____

EXERCISE 4.2   Rating How Safe You Think You Are

The following situations are the same as those listed in the previous exercise. Think again of recent day-to-day situations. *Do not use a traumatic situation for this exercise.* Circle the number for how safe or unsafe you really think you *are* in each of the following situations. For the moment, try to ignore how afraid or safe you emotionally feel. Focus instead on what you rationally think the risk is. If you added situations in the blanks of the Exercise 4.1, add them in the blanks below. Then rate them for how safe you think you are.

Circle

1. Extremely safe	4. Somewhat unsafe
2. Moderately safe	5. Moderately unsafe
3. Somewhat safe	6. Extremely unsafe

How safe am I	Extremely safe					Extremely unsafe
at home with friends or family	1	2	3	4	5	6
at home alone	1	2	3	4	5	6
driving my own car	1	2	3	4	5	6
as a passenger in someone else's car	1	2	3	4	5	6
at work or school	1	2	3	4	5	6
on an airplane, boat, or train	1	2	3	4	5	6
with family outside my home	1	2	3	4	5	6
with friends outside my home	1	2	3	4	5	6
around strangers outside my home	1	2	3	4	5	6
alone outside my home	1	2	3	4	5	6
_____	1	2	3	4	5	6
_____	1	2	3	4	5	6
_____	1	2	3	4	5	6

Do your thoughts and your feelings match for the safest situation? If so, this means that your feelings and thoughts are working together; they are in "sync." But being in sync doesn't necessarily tell you how accurate the message is.

When your thoughts and feelings are not in sync, it is difficult to know which is the more accurate guide to the real risks you face. Do you *feel* danger (i.e., fear, tension) even when you *think* that you are at low risk for harm? Circumstances that used to feel safe may no longer feel that way after trauma.

Do you ever *feel* safe when you objectively *think* you are at a high risk for harm? Do you ever deliberately put yourself in risky situations? If this fits you, you need to be careful. Think before you act, no matter how "safe" a situation feels. Get a second opinion about the level of risk. You may need to think further about this in the exercises that follow.

Do questions about safety provoke strong feelings, intense thoughts, even destructive impulses? Remember, strong feelings and impulses may be from the past but they still need to be respected. Strong negative feelings usually mean you need some self-care and comfort. We will talk more later in this chapter about how to deal with such emotional "triggers." It is important to take good care of yourself when something triggers difficult emotions or memories.

After trauma, it can be difficult to know how accurate your thoughts and feelings are, whether or not they are out of sync. The best way to find out is to look at the evidence outside your thoughts and feelings.

Weighing the Evidence: How Safe Are You Really?

How you think and feel can be distorted by trauma so it is important to pay attention to the outside evidence. If your thoughts and feelings match good, strong evidence, you can probably trust them. If your feelings and thoughts are out of sync, trust what matches the evidence. In Exercise 4.3 we ask you to weigh the evidence for and against how you think and feel in the situations in the previous two exercises. Remember, safety and danger exist together on a continuum. This is as true for facts and evidence as it is for thoughts and feelings.

If your "most safe" and "least safe" situation match in Exercises 4.1 and 4.2, simply list them under (A) and (B), respectively, in Exercise 4.3. If your

EXERCISE 4.3   Weighing the Evidence on How Safe You Really Are

Compare Exercises 4.1 and 4.2. How did your ratings for feeling safe (Exercise 4.1) compare with your rating for thinking you are safe (Exercise 4.2)? Do the most safe and least safe situations from the two exercises match? If so, list them below under (A) and (B), respectively, and then list what facts or evidence support that rating. If your feelings and thoughts about the most safe and least safe situations were different, use the second copy of this exercise provided and do it twice: once to compare your feelings with the evidence, and then a second time to compare your thoughts with the evidence.

A.   List a situation that you rated most *safe* (1 or 2):

_____

What evidence (facts) supports this belief as accurate?

a. _____

b. _____

c. _____

What evidence (facts) supports this belief as not accurate?

a. _____

b. _____

c. _____

B.   List here a situation that you rated most *unsafe* (5 or 6):

_____

What evidence (facts) supports this belief as accurate?

a. _____

b. _____

c. _____

What evidence (facts) supports this belief as not accurate?

a. _____

b. _____

c. _____

**EXERCISE 4.3   Weighing the Evidence on How Safe
You Really Are**

If your ratings for what *feels* like the most safe and least safe situations differed from
your ratings for what you *thought* were the most and least safe situations, use this exercise to examine whichever you didn't look at on page 112.

A.   List a situation that you rated most *safe* (1 or 2):

_____

What evidence (facts) supports this belief as accurate?

a. _____

b. _____

c. _____

What evidence (facts) supports this belief as not accurate?

a. _____

b. _____

c. _____

B.   List here a situation that you rated most *unsafe* (5 or 6):

_____

What evidence (facts) supports this belief as accurate?

a. _____

b. _____

c. _____

What evidence (facts) supports this belief as not accurate?

a. _____

b. _____

c. _____

answers do not match, you might want to do this exercise twice: once to compare your feelings with evidence, and once to compare your thoughts with the evidence.

Exercise 4.3 is designed to give you a sense of how accurate your thoughts and feelings may or may not be. When you finish this exercise, read the next section, which offers tips on how to protect yourself. We recommend you read this whether or not your reactions are accurate.

STRATEGIES FOR PROTECTING YOURSELF

If you have ways to protect yourself, you can make yourself safer. Survivors of trauma often need protection from two different sources. The first is from negative emotions inside themselves; the second is from people and the environment outside themselves. Both can "feel" dangerous and "be" dangerous in some instances.

Protecting Yourself on the Inside

Certain people, places, sounds, smells, sights, or even types of weather may trigger memories, feelings, images, or behaviors associated with the trauma. Answering questions about safety may be a trigger for you. If you believe you are having a trigger reaction at any point as you complete this workbook, *stop*. Take a moment to breathe. However you do it, try to regain some measure of soothing and calm. Being able to do this protects you and gives you some sense of control over the painful or frightening feelings. Having some control may ease your feelings of danger. The following are all ways to protect yourself from negative emotions and thoughts:

- Hold a familiar, safe object.
- Put your feet firmly on the floor; ground yourself in the present.
- Flip to the end of Chapters 1, 2, or 3 and begin doing a relaxation exercise.
- Consult your "Self-Care Plan for Triggers" at the end of the prologue.
- Try to "contain" the feelings or memories (discussed further on).
- Talk to someone.
- Allow yourself to grieve losses.
- Be flexible.

Containment is another coping strategy you can use as emotional self-protection for triggers or similar feelings. It is anything that helps you "contain" or tolerate strong feelings so that they do not overwhelm you and you can attend to this book. Containing strong feelings does not mean eliminating them, but it does mean being able to put them off to the side so that you can focus on something else. If relaxation techniques help you do this, they are containment strategies. Other techniques involve using your imagination. For example, picture yourself putting disturbing memories or feelings in a box, shutting the lid, and pushing the box off to the side. If the traumatic event keeps replaying in your mind, think of it as pictures on a small television screen across the room, or as an imaginary movie within your head and you are simply an audience member. Both of these techniques distance you from the images and feelings, helping to make them less intense.

Protecting Yourself on the Outside

Protecting yourself from the outside sometimes requires different strategies than does protecting yourself on the inside. Most people, however, need ways to do both. The effective coping strategies listed in Chapter 2 can also work to protect you on both the inside and outside. The following are all excellent actions you can take to feel more protected from danger in the outside environment and from other people:

- Learn all you can about what is going to happen.
- Plan ahead.
- Avoid impulsive changes.
- Talk to others who have had similar experiences.
- Take your time.

In the ways of coping checklist in Chapter 2 (pp. 37–41), you checked the kinds of things you usually do when under stress. We then asked you to consider what works for you and what doesn't. In Exercise 4.4, we ask you to list those ways you think would best work to protect yourself from the inside and from the outside. If you wish, you can refer back to your coping checklist in Chapter 2.

EXERCISE 4.4 How Well Do You Protect Yourself?

List the strategies you have used to protect yourself and then rate how effective each one has been. You can refer back to the "Ways I Cope" you checked in Chapter 2.

Circle

1. Extremely effective	4. Fair
2. Very good	5. Poor
3. Good	6. Ineffective

Extremely effective   **Ineffective**

**Ways I protect myself from my
negative feelings, impulses, thoughts:**

1	2	3	4	5	6
1	2	3	4	5	6
1	2	3	4	5	6
1	2	3	4	5	6

Ways I protect myself from others:

1	2	3	4	5	6
1	2	3	4	5	6
1	2	3	4	5	6
1	2	3	4	5	6

Ways I protect myself out in the world:

1	2	3	4	5	6
1	2	3	4	5	6
1	2	3	4	5	6
1	2	3	4	5	6

If you are already using effective strategies, list them. Perhaps this book has given you new ideas for how to protect yourself; if so, list those also. In the blanks under each category in Exercise 4.4, fill in what you now do to protect yourself. Rate how well you feel each strategy works.

Once you've assessed how well you can protect yourself, move on to Exercise 4.5. It asks you to consider how you can best use the most successful strategies you have just identified. Complete Exercise 4.5 now to plan in advance how you can protect yourself when you most need it.

 EXERCISE 4.5   Planning Ahead to Protect Yourself

Consider the most effective ways you have for protecting yourself. Using them, complete the following sentences. If you cannot think of an effective strategy you have already used, complete the sentences with strategies you may not have tried yet but think would be very successful.

If I feel physically unsafe with myself, one way I can protect myself is

_____.

If I feel emotionally unsafe with myself, one way I can protect myself is

_____.

If I feel physically unsafe with others, one way I can protect myself is

_____.

If I feel emotionally unsafe with others, one way I can protect myself is

_____.

If I feel physically unsafe in my environment, one way I can protect myself is

_____.

If I feel emotionally unsafe in my environment, one way I can protect myself is

_____.

DO YOU FEEL SAFE ENOUGH?

In the last section, we asked you to consider ways to protect yourself. Use your effective protection strategies whenever you need to throughout this book and at other times in your daily life. Those strategies can help. They may not, however, make you feel safe enough. By "safe enough," we mean getting your basic needs for safety met. Everyone needs to have a minimum sense of safety. Specifically, you need to believe

- that you are reasonably safe from harm inflicted by yourself, by others, or by the environment
- that people you value are reasonably safe from harm inflicted by yourself, by others, or by the environment

Notice you do not need to believe, you or your loved ones are "always safe," just that they are "reasonably safe." "Reasonably safe" means that the actual level of risk is low enough to be acceptable to you and that you can feel secure and comfortable at that level of risk. There is always *some* level of risk in life, and many people are able to feel safe and comfortable despite it. However, different people have different definitions of what reasonably safe means. What is acceptable risk (and so reasonably safe) to someone else may not be acceptable to you. There is no right or wrong in this. What is important is what safety and risk mean to *you*. If you have a comfortable and accessible sense of safety you may not need to continue working on this issue.

If you are a trauma survivor, you may have difficulty feeling or being safe enough. We want you to respect your thoughts and feelings. Listen to them. Do not try to force yourself to change how you feel. Do not try to ignore how unsafe or afraid you may feel. If you do not feel safe enough, you have reasons for feeling this way. However, you can probably still find safety sometimes in some places. What things or circumstances might be "safe enough" for you even now? The earlier exercises, including self-care activities, should have helped you identify some remaining areas of safety. If your sense of safety can vary from situation to situation, what is it that makes for a safer situation? If you can identify specific things that make you safe, even if very limited, it is possible to use that information to slowly enlarge what is safe for you until you feel safe enough.

When you are ready, Exercise 4.6 (see next page) begins to help you look at the reasons you may have a problem with safety. Be sure that you have and can use tools for protecting yourself before you continue.

TRACKING REACTIONS TO BELIEFS ABOUT SAFETY

Identifying Your Beliefs about Safety

If you have a problem feeling safe enough, the trauma has probably changed a basic belief that you had about safety. You may want to change it back to the way it was before, but this may not be possible. However, you can regain a sense of safety. The first step is to identify what has changed and what you now believe about safety.

The earlier exercises probably reminded you of at least one situation in which you felt a problem with safety, fear, or protecting yourself. Perhaps feelings of fear didn't quite match the facts of something that happened; or perhaps fear kept you from doing something you wanted to be able to do. Think of that situation and then use it with Exercise 4.6. Write down the situation at the start of the exercise; but remember, do not use a traumatic situation for this exercise.

Let's see how Ruby thought through the questions and filled in the blanks for this exercise. She had gone to a therapist because of problems following a trauma. Now she finds herself afraid to talk about the traumatic events that happened to her, even to her therapist in her therapy sessions. Ruby feels like she ought to be able to talk about what happened. But she just can't seem to overcome the fear. This is the situation Ruby uses for the exercise. For the situation description, she writes down

I'm afraid to talk about the trauma in therapy.

The next question asks Ruby what it says about her that she feels unsafe in this situation? She takes time to think about what she just wrote, then she writes

I'm afraid because I might get very upset and lose control. Maybe I won't be able to drive my car out of the parking lot when the session is over.

She thinks about what this statement says about her.

EXERCISE 4.6   Identifying a Belief about Safety

Think of a recent situation in which you had a problem with safety, fear, or protecting yourself. *Do not use a traumatic situation for this exercise.* Did you rate any situations in the earlier exercises as unsafe? Describe a specific situation in the first space below. Then write what you think that situation says about you. What does it mean that you thought the situation unsafe? After you write down a response, look at what you just wrote. Then write what *that* says about you. Continue answering the questions by looking at your immediately preceding answers.

Situation:

_____

_____

What does this say or mean about me?

_____

_____

_____

Looking at what I just wrote, what does *that* say or mean about me?

_____

_____

_____

What does *that*, in turn, say or mean about me?

_____

_____

_____

Looking at all the above, can I drawn any conclusions about myself?

_____

_____

_____

Adapted with permission from Dennis Greenberger and Christine Padesky. *Mind Over Mood: Change How You Feel by Changing the Way You Think.* New York: Guilford Press, 1995.

I'm afraid because I have to look out for a lot of stuff. If I can't, who is going to do it for me?

Then she thinks, what does this mean? She writes

I am very responsible; I have to be.

Thinking about this, she writes:

I'm not sure this therapist can help me if I get too upset.

Reading through the entire exercise, she now thinks about what it says about her and safety:

Talking about the trauma can make me lose control and that feels very danger-ous. If I can't count on myself, I'm not sure I can count on the therapist to help.

Ruby looked at this exercise and wondered how her answers could pos-sibly help her. She felt just as stuck as before. She couldn't see anything new or helpful in what she'd written, but she was a step ahead of herself. She was looking at her answers for clues on how to change. This exercise, however, was designed to help Ruby understand how she is *now*. Knowing this will help her know better what to do to move forward. For Ruby this means un-derstanding *why* she feels and thinks she is unsafe in the situation. Ruby looked again at what she had written in the exercise. Her goal now was sim-ply to see what she is saying. To do this, she must avoid judging or evaluating what she's written. There is a place for evaluating, but it's not here. Ruby has written that staying safe means staying in control of herself. This makes sense. Feeling out of control and unable to function *is* frighten-ing. This fear is made stronger by her belief that she can't really count on her therapist. In other words, safety for Ruby means feeling in control of herself. It is also connected to being able to trust another. If she cannot stay in con-trol and she cannot trust her therapist, then she may be right to protect her-self by not talking about the trauma. This surprised Ruby. She had assumed that the way she felt and behaved must be a problem. It had not occurred to her that this could also be a good thing, helping her to stay safe. Later Ruby found it helpful when she looked at Chapters 5 and 6 on control and trust. But for now, Ruby's next step is to think more about how her belief both helps her and hinders her.

Evaluating How a Belief Helps and Hinders You

After trauma, most people feel different. Trauma changes things. Ruby needs to pay attention to her feelings of being unsafe. Are her feelings accurate in the present or are they about the past? Are her beliefs helping her more than getting in her way? Her beliefs about safety since the trauma have caused her problems. Ruby needs to think about these questions before she does anything to change her behavior or her beliefs one way or the other. Exercise 4.7 helps you look systematically at how a particular belief helps and hinders you. The answers may not be as clear-cut as you think. For each question, Ruby could not simply say yes or no. She needed to think about where on a scale, between all and nothing, her answers fell.

Look at the belief on the last line of Exercise 4.6 that you just finished. Then answer the questions in Exercise 4.7. When you finish, look at your overall evaluation of the belief. Perhaps the belief has some drawbacks, but overall it is helpful. Perhaps it has some positive aspects but many drawbacks. On the whole, are your answers more toward positive or negative? If the belief tends to hinder you more than help, you might want to consider how accurate it really is. You might want to keep an open mind about this belief and pay attention to the evidence.

Pinpointing Problem Areas to Think Through Further

We hope you have been able to identify at least one underlying belief about safety; however, you certainly have more than just one. Most people have many different beliefs about any important need. If you have identified a belief that may be causing you problems, consider thinking through that belief further. The actual work of thinking through the belief does not need to be done quickly or right now. Go at your own pace. For the moment, we want only to take stock of the information you have gathered so far.

Do you worry a lot about safety for yourself or others? If so, where do you see danger? Is it from other people? From the physical environment? From inside yourself? Do your thoughts, feelings, and impulses ever frighten you? If so, do you think you could sometimes be a danger to yourself or others? How likely are you to act on dangers that come from within you? Can you control those dangers or do you think you could hurt yourself or another? If you answer yes to these questions, it is essential that you talk with

EXERCISE 4.7 How Does This Belief Help and Hinder Me?

Most beliefs have both advantages and disadvantages. Consider those for the belief you identified in Exercise 4.6. Write down the belief in the space below then circle how helpful or hindering the belief is for each question.

Belief:

_____

Circle

1. Extremely helpful	4. Not at all helpful
2. Very helpful	5. Gets in my way
3. Moderately helpful	6. Gets in my way a lot

	Extremely helpful			Gets in my way a lot		
1. How helpful is this belief?	1	2	3	4	5	6
2. How calming is this belief?	1	2	3	4	5	6
3. How flexible is this belief?	1	2	3	4	5	6
4. How safe does this belief make me feel?	1	2	3	4	5	6
5. Does this belief help me understand myself?	1	2	3	4	5	6
6. Does this belief give me hope?	1	2	3	4	5	6
7. How essential is the belief to my survival?	1	2	3	4	5	6
8. How well does this belief help me cope?	1	2	3	4	5	6
9. Does this belief help me make sense of the world?	1	2	3	4	5	6
10. Does this belief help me make decisions?	1	2	3	4	5	6
11. Does this belief help me know what I need for myself?	1	2	3	4	5	6

a supportive person you trust and get some help. Doing this does not mean you must be weak or crazy; it reflects what you learned from your experiences.

If you feel you do have a problem with safety, what particular areas present problems for you? Take a look at your answers to the above questions and for the seven exercises you have completed so far. Check below any or all of the items that are relevant to you. You may have more than one check per question.

Whom are you afraid for (who might be hurt)?

Yourself _____   People close to you _____

What are you afraid of (from where would the danger come)?

Your emotions _____   Your actions _____   Other people's emotions _____

Other people's actions _____   The physical environment _____

If you have checked any of the above items, you could use that item to continue thinking about safety when you are ready.

Time Out for Self-Care

It is very important to be good to yourself, to learn ways to soothe and comfort yourself. Take a few minutes now to do that. Say the following affirmations about safety to yourself.

I have the right to be safe in my world.

I have access to a safe place in my world.

The people I love have a right to be safe in the world.

Can you think of others?

Taking Stock

Pause now to consider what you need and want. Do you want to continue working on safety issues? If you would like to put this work aside for now, feel free to do so. If you prefer to move on to other issues right now, feel free to do that. Exercise 4.8 asks you take stock of where you are in your work on safety. Fill this out as a record, then move on to do whatever you need to do for yourself right now.

∞ EXERCISE 4.8   Taking Stock of Your Work on Safety

Consider what you think and feel right now. Do you wish take a break from this work? Do you wish to continue? Please check the statement that describes your situation right now.

_____ 1. My beliefs about my own physical and emotional safety are fine. I do not need to think them through further. I feel as safe as I need to feel.

_____ 2. My beliefs about the safety of others are fine. I do not need to think them through further. The people about whom I care are as safe as I need them to be.

_____ 3. There are ways that I might not be safe enough, but I do not wish to work further now on what safety means to me. I can come back to work on this chapter whenever I feel ready.

_____ 4. The people about whom I care might not be safe enough, but I do not wish to work further in this chapter now. I can come back to this work whenever I feel ready.

_____ 5. I am beginning to think about why some of my beliefs about safety do not work. I can continue working on these beliefs, but I want to move slowly and carefully. I can stop this work at any time.

_____ 6. I am ready to think through a belief about safety.

If you checked 5 or 6 above, write down here any beliefs that you may wish to work on, whether at sometime in the future or now.

_____

_____

_____

_____

_____

_____

THINKING THROUGH A BELIEF ABOUT SAFETY

The rest of this chapter helps you look at the beliefs you have about safety in more detail. The exercises ask you to think about feeling unsafe, feeling fear, and what to do when you feel in danger. Remember to protect yourself as you do these exercises. *Do not use a traumatic situation for any of these exercises.* Stop if you feel emotionally overwhelmed or if memories of the trauma are triggered.

Choosing Beliefs to Work On

Make a list below of the beliefs you have identified so far that you would like to think through more completely. Perhaps you have none, or only one. Perhaps you have several. Write down any that you have:

_____

_____

_____

For each of the above beliefs, complete Exercise 4.9 (beginning on page 128). Make extra copies of the blank form if you wish. Remember that thinking through just one belief takes time. It requires consideration of many different things. As we explained earlier, the questions in this next exercise take you through the following steps:

- Sort out the facts of what happened.
- Sort out the meaning the facts have for you.
- Identify the underlying belief.
- Evaluate the pros and cons of the belief.
- Imagine alternative meanings for the same facts.
- Evaluate the pros and cons of the alternative meanings.
- Consider how to check the accuracy of these beliefs.
- Put the process in perspective.

Sort Out the Facts, Sort Out the Meaning, Identify the Belief

Exercise 4.9 starts by asking you to write down the belief you wish to think through. Think then of a particular situation in which that belief may have been a problem. It is fine to use the same situation you used to identify the belief. Describe the "facts" of what happened in that situation. How did you interpret those facts? Based on your interpretation, what do you think you believe about safety? If you have trouble identifying a belief at this point, use Exercise 4.7 to identify a belief.

Evaluate the Pros and Cons of the Belief

Once you have identified the belief, we ask you to evaluate it by looking at it in a number of different ways. How old is this belief? If it is recent, it will be easier to change than if it comes from your childhood. How does the belief help you or hinder you? In other words, do you want to change it? or do the advantages outweigh the disadvantages?

Imagine Alternative Meanings for the Same Facts

Even when the belief has advantages, can you think of other ways the facts could be interpreted? Can you think of at least one other alternative meaning the facts could have?

Evaluate the Pros and Cons of the Alternative Meaning

Alternative meanings will also have pros and cons. How do the advantages and disadvantages stack up compared to the existing belief? Is there an alternative meaning that fits the facts well but has more advantages than your old belief?

Consider How to Check the Accuracy of These Beliefs

As a mental exercise consider how you might collect evidence on the accuracy of the belief and the alternative meaning. We do not want you to actually do anything; we are asking only that you try to imagine one or two ways you could find evidence for or against your two interpretations of the facts.

The question of checking or testing beliefs needs to be carefully thought through. There is a risk involved and your safety is the priority. You

EXERCISE 4.9   Steps for Thinking Through a Belief about Trust of Self or Others

The belief you wish to think through:

_____

Sort Out the Facts of What Happened

Think of a particular situation in which this belief may have been a problem. You can use the same situation you used to identify the belief, or use another situation in which you worried about your own safety or that of people about whom you care. Describe the facts. What happened? What was the sequence of events?

Sort Out the Meaning the Facts Have for You

How did you interpret this situation? What did it mean to you?

Identify the Underlying Belief

What lesson did you draw from it about yourself? About other people?

When did you start believing this about yourself or others? Was this incident the first time? If not, when and how do you remember first learning this lesson?

Evaluate the Pros and Cons of the Belief

How does believing this make you feel about yourself or others? What does it make you think about yourself or others?

How does believing this help you or protect you?

How does believing this hold you back or get in your way?

Imagine Alternative Meanings for the Same Facts

Look back at your description of what happened (the first question above). Are there other ways to interpret what happened? What else could the situation mean? Is there an alternative meaning that would fit the facts of what happened? If so, what is it?

Evaluate the Pros and Cons of the Alternative Meaning

What positive feelings do you have when you think about this alternative meaning?

What negative feelings do you have when you think about this alternative meaning?

Consider How to Check the Accuracy of These Beliefs

How could you test to see whether or not your belief is true?

How high is the risk if you test the truth of what you believe? How dangerous would it be?

What good things might happen if you test the truth of what you believe?

Put the Process in Perspective

Will testing the belief matter 10 years from now? Would it help or hinder you in the future?

may feel right now that any risk is too big. Respect that feeling. However, not all risks are big. There may be other small, low-risk ways to collect evidence on a belief. Later in this chapter, in Exercise 4.12, we will ask you to think in terms of "baby steps" for testing a belief. You have probably already done one of those steps, which is to pay attention to the evidence that you see around you as you go about your normal activities.

Put the Process in Perspective

It can be frightening to think of taking any kind of risk, especially when the basic concern is safety. It is important to remember, however, that you do not have to take any action right now. Many readers will not be ready to consider checking evidence on safety until after they read through the rest of the book. When the idea of collecting evidence begins to seem like a possibility, it can help to consider the long-term advantages and disadvantages. How much will it matter in 10 years if you check out the evidence of your belief? What if you do check it and it's wrong? If the long-term advantages begin to outweigh the short-term disadvantages, such as the risk, then you might be ready to think further.

WEIGHING THE EVIDENCE ON BELIEFS ABOUT SAFETY

Your responses to thinking through a belief in Exercise 4.9 may bring you a long way or only a little way toward rethinking what you believe about safety. Even if you think you have logically figured out some things, you may not believe or feel it. Believing in and feeling safe enough—when you don't now—takes time. It takes time for the weight of evidence to accumulate and your beliefs to accommodate to that evidence. Beliefs about safety, in particular, are difficult to change. Take your time. When you feel ready to work further on safety, you can help move the process forward by paying attention to the evidence in a systematic way.

Weigh the Evidence on the Existing Belief

If there is a belief you wish you could change, or feel differently about, keep an open mind about its accuracy and begin to collect evidence. Start by collecting the evidence you *already* have. What facts do your present experience and recent memory give you? In Exercise 4.10 (see next page), we want you to list the actions, events, or facts that support the belief's accuracy and those that do not. Remember that feelings and thoughts are not facts. Interpretations and meanings are not facts either, although they are based on facts. Facts are what you can see, hear, touch, taste, and smell. They can be something you or another person says, or actions you perform or witness.

After you have listed the available evidence, rate how strongly you hold the belief. Be honest. You probably wouldn't need to do this exercise unless the weight of the current evidence was in favor of the belief, even though you wish it were otherwise.

Weigh the Evidence on an Alternative Meaning

In Exercise 4.9, we asked you to think of other ways to interpret the facts of a situation. Could you think of anything? Did it have more advantages than what you now believe? Do you wish you could believe the alternative interpretation, even though you may not be able to right now? Regardless of what you think or feel about this alternative meaning, list the objective evidence for and against its accuracy by completing Exercise 4.11 (see page 133). It is the same exercise you just completed for the existing belief. How well does the alternative interpretation match the evidence? Next, rate how strongly you believe in the accuracy of this alternative meaning.

If you are looking for dramatic changes the first time you rate the old and new beliefs, you will probably be disappointed. Change takes time and you are only starting to think about the process. These exercises show where you are now. As you collect new evidence your beliefs should slowly change. You can find out if they are changing by coming back to these exercises later and again rating the strength of your beliefs as well as possibly adding to the lists of evidence reflecting the degree of accuracy of the beliefs.

Collect New Evidence on Safety

In Chapter 3, we talked about Carol. She was able to think of some low-risk ways to check her belief that terrible things would happen if she expressed a feeling. The first four ways of collecting evidence consisted simply of paying attention to particular things that were already happening. This may sound

EXERCISE 4.10   What Evidence Do I Have about the Existing Belief?

What evidence do you already have about the accuracy of your existing belief? What facts, words, or actions support the belief? What facts, words, or actions indicate the belief is inaccurate? Write those down below.

Belief: _____

What facts or evidence support this belief as accurate?

1. _____

2. _____

3. _____

What facts or evidence indicate this belief is not accurate?

1. _____

2. _____

3. _____

How sure are you that this belief is accurate? Mark how sure on the following scale. Use the second evaluation scale later to check on changes in your beliefs in light of new evidence.

Date: _____

Accurate   Inaccurate

_____

100%   50%   0%

Date: _____

Accurate   Inaccurate

_____

100%   50%   0%

**EXERCISE 4.11   What Evidence Do I Have
about the Alternative Meaning?**

What evidence do you already have about the accuracy of the alternative meaning?
What facts, words, or actions support the alternative meaning? What facts, words, or
actions indicate the alternative meaning is inaccurate? Write those down below.

Alternative meaning: _____

What facts or evidence support this interpretation as accurate?

1. _____
2. _____
3. _____

What facts or evidence indicate this interpretation is not accurate?

1. _____
2. _____
3. _____

How sure are you that this interpretation is accurate? Mark how sure on the following
scale. Use the second evaluation scale later to check on changes in your beliefs in light
of new evidence.

Date: _____

Accurate   Inaccurate

_____

100%   50%   0%

Date: _____

Accurate   Inaccurate

_____

100%   50%   0%

too easy to be of help, but it is likely there is much evidence you don't see. This is particularly true of any evidence that contradicts your old beliefs. Collecting evidence on a belief means making a real effort to see the facts and evidence without leaping to any conclusions.

Think now about a belief you hold about yourself or other people that you would like to check out. The idea of testing a belief probably feels risky. Remember, it is only an idea. We do not want you to do anything until you have thought carefully about it and you have a plan for low-risk methods of collecting evidence.

Brainstorm Ideas for Collecting Evidence

Before you do anything, you need lots of ideas for how to stay safe while collecting evidence. One way to gather ideas is to brainstorm. You can use Exercise 4.12 or use a blank piece of paper. Write down *all* the ideas that come into your head no matter how unlikely, impractical, or silly they seem. Try to think of as many low-risk methods as possible. Examples of low-risk methods include the following:

1. Notice or observe events or actions and the people acting.
2. Watch other people's reactions to the event or action.
3. Notice when you yourself are already carrying out actions that produce evidence about your belief.
4. Ask friends questions about their reactions.
5. When it feels safe enough, take a small action with a safe friend and see how the friend reacts to you.

Rank Ideas by Lowest Risk First

The next step is to consider the level of risk involved in the ideas you have brainstormed. For example, after his car accident Kirk felt unsafe and at risk outside his house. Being outside anywhere felt risky. But some places felt riskier than others. For example, driving a car seemed most risky. Although walking down the street to a neighborhood store also felt risky, it was less so. You may want to look back to the beginning of this chapter. How did you fill out Exercise 4.1, "Rating How Safe You Feel"? You probably felt variations

EXERCISE 4.12   Brainstorm Ideas for Collecting Evidence on a Belief

Create a list of rough ideas for collecting evidence on a belief. The goal is to come up with some low-risk ways to collect evidence, but be prepared that the first ideas you have may be high risk. Write them down to get them out of the way. You do not need to carry out *any* of the ideas you write down. You will screen these ideas later and discard any you choose. Begin by writing down a belief and an alternative interpretation on which you want to collect evidence. In the blank space below write down any and all ideas that come to mind for how to do this.

Belief: _____

Alternative interpretation: _____

of risk depending on the situations in the exercise. Use those answers to help you consider that different situations can have different levels of risk for you.

When you feel ready, begin to fill out Exercise 4.13. Begin by writing the belief you wish to test at the top. Then think of very specific but small efforts you can make to test a belief. Feel free to borrow from Tina's steps, which were

Least Feared Actions/Observations

pay attention to how other people act, what they do, on this issue

pay attention to how other people respond to these actions

pay attention to how you already do this yourself, even slightly

pay attention to how other people respond when you do this yourself

ask a trusted friend how he or she feels when you do this

try doing the action just a little more with a trusted friend then asking his or her reaction

try the action with another friend

ask the friend how he or she reacted

try the action with strangers

try the action with people in authority over you

Most Feared Actions/Observations

The act of making the list can be helpful by itself without your further action. Making this list does not commit you to do any of these steps. You are free to choose not to take any of the steps. If you choose to carry any of them out, do so only when you feel ready and then move at a pace that is most comfortable for you.

Carry Out the Lowest Risk Ways to Collect Evidence

If you decide to take a small step to test a belief, start with the least feared, lowest risk action on the list. Then keep doing it for awhile. Let the evidence from that step accumulate over some time. For example, you could decide to try the first step for one week. During that week, at the end of each day,

EXERCISE 4.13   Baby Steps for Testing a Belief about Safety

In the first blanks below, write down the belief you are thinking of testing and an alternative interpretaion. When you have brainstormed ideas for possible ways to collect evidence on a belief, rank those ideas by risk, starting with the lowest risk ways. List only ways that are within a reasonable risk. Do not list any high-risk ways to collect evidence.

Belief: _____

Alternative interpretation: _____

Least Feared Actions/Observations

_____

_____

_____

_____

_____

_____

_____

_____

_____

_____

Most Feared Actions/Observations

write down any evidence for and against the belief that you have collected. After a week, try rating the belief again. How sure are you now that your belief is accurate? Has your rating changed since the first time you rated your belief, even if only a little bit? Notice if there's any shift but don't expect to draw any conclusions yet. Continue to keep an open mind.

How risky does that first step feel after you have done it for a week? It probably will feel less risky over time, if you give it enough time. Do the first step for a second week if the next step feels too risky for you; but when you feel comfortable with the level of risk in the next step, try that for a week. As you feel ready and comfortable, slowly try each next step for testing the belief. In this way, the evidence will accumulate and your beliefs about safety will change to accommodate the weight of the evidence.

SUMMARIZING YOUR WORK ON SAFETY

Move on from this chapter when you wish. Come back to it when you feel ready. In the meantime, make a record of your work so far. Fill out as much of Exercise 4.14 as you can and date it.

Safety is a basic need. It is the most important need that you may have right now. Whatever your beliefs about safety are now, they probably help you in some ways. They may also put you at risk or prevent you from healing and living fully. Do you believe you are safe without first checking the evidence or considering the risk? If so, you leave yourself vulnerable to further harm. Do you believe that safety and risk cannot coexist? If so, your belief can stunt your growth and create difficulties with trust and intimacy. After trauma, you may not know anymore what you believe. This is part of the problem, but it also points the way to the solution.

The path back to safety begins with understanding where you are right now. What do you think, feel, and believe it means to be safe? When you begin to make your beliefs conscious and to put them into words, you begin to regain some personal power. You can then consider what else safety might mean and understand better what you need in order to be safe. We cannot tell you what to believe, but you do not have to let the trauma be your only guide. Be open to all the evidence and let the weight of it guide you toward what you can believe in again.

As you end this chapter, remember how it feels to be safe, secure, protected. Remember how it feels to know those close to you are safe from harm. If you know how these things feel, you can come to feel it again safely.

EXERCISE 4.14   Summarizing Your Work on Safety

I have identified the following beliefs about safety:

I can think of the following alternative meanings:

I have already carried out the following steps (mark with X); or I would like in the future to carry out the following steps (mark with *):

_____ Make a list of what evidence might confirm and/or contradict the existing belief.

_____ Organize the list of evidence from least feared/least risky to collect. to most feared/most risky to collect.

_____ Carry out the least feared/least risky way to collect evidence.

_____ Keep a record of the evidence collected—both pro and con.

List here any evidence collected—what did you see or do, and how did it turn out? Continue adding to this list over time as you become aware of additional evidence.

CHAPTER FIVE

WHAT DOES IT MEAN TO TRUST?

YOUR NEED FOR TRUST: The need to rely on your own judgment; the need to rely on others.

JUST TRUST YOURSELF, then you will know how to live.

—Goethe, *Faust*

HOW TRUST CAN BE AN ISSUE AFTER TRAUMA

Trust and safety are related. When you can trust yourself and others, it helps you feel safer in the world. When others prove themselves trustworthy, you feel more secure and less alone. When you trust yourself, you feel confident and less at risk. However, it can be difficult to trust after trauma. During traumatic events something important that you trusted may have proved unreliable. This can shatter a sense of trust just as it can shatter a sense of safety.

We all need some sense of trust in ourselves and in others. We need to be able to rely on our own judgment, have confidence in our own abilities, and trust our gut instincts. We also need to be able to count on other people to be there for us when we need them, whether the need is for a hammer, a cup of sugar, or a confidante.

Trusting Others

When trauma involves violence or negligence by another person, trust in others can become an issue. How can you trust other people if they have put you in danger?

❧ *Greg grew up in a household filled with violence. His father constantly carried a loaded gun. When drinking, he often pointed it at Greg's head. Greg's brother frequently hit Greg after being disciplined by their father. Greg learned that the members of his family could not be trusted to be loving and kind. His need to trust others was denied. Greg learned that it was best never to trust.*

For Greg, trust and safety are very intertwined. Greg cannot trust others to respect his need for safety. At an essential level, trusting others is about believing they will not hurt you. It doesn't take repeated traumas to disrupt a sense of trust in others. It can happen even if you have experienced a single traumatic event.

❧ *Betty worked in the business office of a famous resort. As the office was closing one night, a young man came into the office and demanded the day's receipts. The man was agitated. He paced back and forth as he made his demands, unaware that there were other employees still in the office. Betty was eager to give him the money to make him go away. Suddenly, another employee burst into the room and struggled with the robber. A gun went off. The young employee was shot in the chest. He fell to the floor and died shortly after. The robber took the money and fled but was later caught. Betty continues to work at the same place. An alarm system and hidden cameras now guard the office. This helps her feel safer but she still finds it difficult to trust others. She is hypervigilant—on guard—when anyone she doesn't know approaches the office.*

Betty assumed that she was safe from the violence and crime that happens in our society. She trusted that no one would harm her at work. The robbery taught Betty a difficult truth: Neither trust nor safety are 100 percent reliable. Because the danger during the robbery was so great, Betty feels she must keep her risk to an absolute minimum. She now fears that anyone might harm her at work at any time. This caution carries a price. She had enjoyed working at the resort because she met people from around the country. Now she is not as relaxed and friendly as she was before. She limits her contacts during the workday and is not enjoying her work as much.

Trusting Ourselves

Trauma can disrupt a sense of trust in yourself as well as in others. Many traumatized people blame themselves for the terrible things that happened to them. They think "I should have fought harder," "I shouldn't have been walking alone," or "I should have known that was going to happen." These normal thoughts can leave them feeling mistrustful about themselves. They begin to question their decisions and doubt their gut feelings.

> ❋ *Deep down Rachel blamed herself for the rape. She felt she should have known better. When she went on dates after the assault, she sometimes felt uneasy. She chalked up these feelings to leftover fear from her horrible experience. She ignored the knots in her stomach she sometimes got with other men.*

Rachel's feelings of uneasiness were internal messages from herself, but she did not trust herself enough to pay attention to them. She assumed the feelings were all from the past and had nothing to do with the present. As we saw earlier, this is sometimes true, but sometimes it's not true. Rachel, however, didn't think through her feelings; she just ignored them. Ignoring such feelings makes it hard for her to distinguish comfortable from uncomfortable, safe from unsafe situations. This, in turn, makes it difficult for her to protect and care for herself. Rachel is not to blame for the rape, but it has undermined her trust in herself. Lack of trust in yourself following trauma can increase your risk for further victimization. This is one reason it is so important to look at your sense of trust following trauma.

Trauma Survivors Speak about Trust

• Trust is being able to believe in what people say—that they won't lie to me, that I can count on their doing what they say they are going to do and not do what is unexpected. Trust is believing that people won't harm me intentionally.

• Trust means opening up little by little. Trust is learned; it is not being a victim.

• The child I was—is no more. The trust I had—is no more. The good memories—are no more; if ever they were—What's left? An adult without the normal experiences of childhood. An adult who trusts one person right now and is frightened by it.

• Trust isn't a topic I'm entirely comfortable with. For one thing, I'm not sure I know how to define trust. Some things are easy to trust, like the world will keep on spinning or the sun will come up. I don't spend a lot of time worrying about that. Those are the laws of nature, I guess. But people are another matter. The one thing I know about people is that they will only care about me if I'm being who they want me to be when they want me to be, and where and how they want me to be. If I step out of line or don't measure up, they will walk away every time. . . . So if I want to be able to trust and depend on someone, I'd better be what they want me to be.

WHAT CAN TRUST MEAN?

After experiencing a crime, as Betty or Rachel did, it can be difficult to know whether trust is possible. When and how might you begin to trust again? For Rachel, the rape survivor, being trustworthy had meant being consistent, reliable, available, honest, and following through with what you say. Trust meant counting on others to respect her physical and emotional boundaries. She had learned the hard lesson that not everyone can be counted on for these things. In the aftermath of trauma, the safest reaction may be to trust nothing and no one. Even doing this, however, cannot guarantee safety. There is no absolute safety; nor is trust absolute. People are imperfect. Even well-intentioned, reliable people sometimes fail when you need to count on them. Even consistent people aren't consistent 100 percent of the time. What, then, does it mean to trust? How can you know when it is or isn't safe to trust?

Trust is a judgment that you make about yourself, another person, or a thing based on your experience and your need. It isn't just any judgment; it is one you depend on in some way. It concerns something that you need. You need your car to start in the morning; it's important. How much do you trust it to start? Your trust in the car probably isn't blind. Blind trust is high risk; it is trusting on the basis of luck or chance and wishing that you will get what you need. Trust, however, is usually earned. If you trust your car to start, it probably has been reliable in the past. Your sense of trust is based on evidence.

Trusting often involves counting on people or things to behave in the future as they've behaved in the past. This is why consistency and reliability are important aspects of trust. The more consistent someone is, the more confidently you can usually count on them. This is why we speak of "earning" someone's trust. It means people give us evidence in their past behavior that we can count on them over time. When you trust a person, it is usually because you have some evidence or experience of their past behavior. This holds for your trust in yourself as well. If your past decisions have consistently turned out well, you will tend to trust your decision-making ability. However, no one can predict the future. The decision to trust can never be made with absolute certainty. There is always some risk. At any point, safety and danger will be mixed together in varying proportions, so too will be trust and disappointment.

How much or how little evidence does it take before you feel comfortable trusting? If you need iron-clad proof you will probably not feel comfortable trusting anything or anybody. However, trusting a coworker to give you a ride to work does not mean you must trust her in other ways, for other things, or even at other times. Trust is not all or nothing. It has many variations and degrees.

Trust can mean different things based on what it is you are counting on. Are you trusting someone's honesty? reliability? understanding? Or is your trust much more specific such as trusting that the chef in a restaurant can, in fact, cook. Perhaps the chef cannot cook and you can't eat the food. You are left without dinner, something you need. Fortunately, the consequence of this disappointment can be remedied more easily than can some other kinds of disappointment.

It is possible to both trust and distrust the same person but for different things. You may highly trust a friend's sense of direction but not at all trust his taste in clothes. Your overall sense of trust in this friend may change depending on the situation. Is he your traveling companion or your shopping companion? What do you need from yourself, or from another in a particular situation? How bad will the consequences be if your trust fails? How strong is your need?

You may not be aware of it, but we often automatically weigh the pros and cons when deciding whether or not to trust. The weighing of pros and cons can be simple and straightforward, or it can get quite complicated. The degree of risk is an important factor. You might trust a person enough to ask for a ride to work but not enough to confide your personal problems. Both are ways of trusting, but they do not involve the same level of risk. The consequences of trust's failure will be quite different depending on whether it is a promised ride that falls through or a promise of intimacy, safety, or one of the other basic needs discussed in this book.

There may be situations in which you need to trust when you would rather not. Perhaps your car breaks down and you must decide whether to accept help from another, unknown, driver. Accepting the help requires some level of trust. Accepting the help also means some level of risk. When both the risk and the need are high, the degree of trust may be very thin and fragile. The decision to trust or not will come out of a weighing of the following factors:

- *The degree of your need.* How badly do you need this? What are the consequences if you don't get what you need right now?

- *The degree of risk.* What will be the consequences if your trust in the person fails?

- *Your own past experiences.* For example, do you know this person, this kind of situation? What is your experience in making these decisions? What have you learned about trust from past experiences?

- *Any other information and evidence you might be able to gather.* What are the immediate circumstances? Is it day or night? Are other people around? What can you tell about the person from how they appear and behave? What are your gut instincts about this person?

Fragile trust is still trust; uncertain trust is still trust; limited trust is still trust. Trust can involve varying degrees of comfort and confidence. When we try something for the first time, it often involves some minimal trust in our abilities. We may not be confident about those abilities, however, until they prove themselves trustworthy. Trust takes time. It comes out of experience and evidence. Something "trustworthy" is by definition something that has stood a test of time. A trusty car is one that has a history of starting when it is needed. But there was always a first time, before you knew how much you really could trust your car.

When trust fails, it can be for different reasons and mean different things. At a minimum, when trust fails, you are left with having to get a need met in some other way or not at all. When the need is emotional, the risk for hurt can be great. When we depend on other people to meet some of our emotional needs, we reveal parts of ourselves we may usually keep private. To receive emotional comfort, we usually have to reveal our emotional upset. We trust the person not to misuse the information or repeat it to others. Some trauma survivors have learned the hard way that it is not always safe to trust others with too much information about themselves. You may be reluctant to say much about yourself to others. Perhaps you do not tell the truth when answering questions about yourself.

Trusting others to keep their word is another very important part of trust. Survivors of repeated trauma can learn over time that people cannot be trusted in this way. You may have experiences with people who did not keep promises they made to you. Some people do not take their promises seriously. Perhaps they had good intentions, but they could not, in the end, come through for you. Unintended disappointments of trust happen because people are imperfect. This can be painful, but a much more severe disappointment is intentional betrayal—when another person seems to have intended harm. When trauma involves intentional harm, such as in a crime or abuse, trust can totally collapse into feeling betrayed.

If trauma has disrupted your sense of trust, the risk of trusting may seem too great. You may feel it is best not to trust yourself or anyone again. You may feel incapable of trusting, even though you may wish you could. But you probably still have some level of trust working for you, even if limited. There are still things and perhaps people you can count on some, if not most, of the time. However, it is reasonable after trauma to want new evidence that people and things can still be trustworthy. Your posttrauma needs can challenge or disrupt some of your existing relationships. Your needs may have changed and those close to you may not be able to support you in the ways you need right now. You may find that you can trust some people with your feelings and thoughts about the trauma. But you may need to protect these vulnerable parts of yourself in other relationships.

To begin to trust again, you need to be open to the weight of the evidence. This chapter is designed to help you begin to gather the evidence, while keeping your risk low.

WHAT DOES TRUST MEAN TO YOU?

In the previous section, we described some of the many meanings that trust can have. These meanings can change depending on who, what, or how much you are trusting. Think about the different aspects of trust described so far in this chapter, then try to answer the following questions. We ask you to think first specifically about trusting yourself, then we ask you about trusting others.

Trusting Yourself

Do you have qualities, skills, or abilities you feel you can rely on? What are they?

Do you see yourself as independent? In other words, do you feel generally confident when on your own and handling things by yourself?

Do you find it difficult to make a choice when you must decide something?

Do you think you make generally good decisions?

Do you tend to keep promises? What does it mean to you when you don't keep a promise?

Do you consider yourself to be a trustworthy person? Why?

When we encounter something for the first time, we occasionally have an immediate gut reaction; this can be called intuition. We may immediately like or dislike a person without quite knowing why. We may feel comfortable or uneasy, again without being able to say why. Have you ever noticed having immediate gut reactions to a person or situation?

If you remember having such reactions, what did you do with them? Did you

____ dismiss them right away and not take them seriously?

____ trust them enough to watch for evidence about their accuracy?

____ trust them enough to act on them immediately?

Trusting Others

What characteristics make another person trustworthy to you?

Do you have friends, family, neighbors, coworkers, church members, and/or a therapist whom you trust? You may have only one or two persons whom you most trust or you may have many people. List the people you trust most in your life. What is it that makes each of them trustworthy? For what can you count on them?

1. _____

2. _____

3. _____

4. _____

5. _____

6. _____

Taken together, the people you have listed create a support system for you. Do you feel you have a support system available to you?

Have you ever asked any of the people you listed above for help?

When do you ask others for help?

____ for help with practical problems and tasks
____ for help with emotional problems and comfort
____ other times

How do you feel when you have to ask for help?

How do you decide when it's probably all right to trust someone, and when it's probably not all right?

Do you come to trust people slowly, quickly, or all at once?

Have others broken promises to you? What promises?

Do you sometimes feel you cannot trust anyone? Do you feel that people always let you down? In what specific situations have you felt this?

Have you ever been surprised that a person is more trustworthy than you expected?

Trusting means depending on someone for something. If you have been let down, abandoned, or betrayed, you may now protect yourself from being hurt by trusting no one. You may try to depend on no one but yourself. It is valuable and important to be able to rely on yourself, but it is lonely, and ultimately impossible, to be totally independent. You may, however, feel you have little or no choice if experience has taught you never to count on other people. Trusting, having to depend on others, can feel extremely uncomfortable, even dangerous. You may think that depending on anyone means being completely dependent. The words dependence and dependent imply a state of helplessness, of having no choice but to rely on others for what is needed. Dependence implies a loss of control over one's own life. Babies are completely dependent on others for the basic necessities of life. The failure of others to meet these needs has life and death consequences for the baby. Most adults, however, are neither totally helpless and dependent nor totally independent and alone. The basic need for trust can be satisfied without requiring complete dependence and helplessness. It is highly risky to trust in this complete and total way. Looking at how you feel about dependence and independence can help you think through the need to trust.

Are you self-sufficient? In other words, for which needs can you rely on yourself to meet? Specifically what are those needs ?

What feelings do you have when you feel independent?

How do you feel when you have to depend on another person?

What does it mean to you to be dependent?

SORTING OUT FACTS ABOUT TRUST FROM REACTIONS: SHADES OF GRAY

How have you answered the above questions? Do you trust your decisions, your instincts, your abilities? Do you think you must be highly competent or skilled to rely on yourself for anything? Do you automatically assume a person is completely trustworthy whether or not you know much about him or her? Do you think that trusting people means you must trust them completely about everything? Do you think that if you can't totally trust someone then you cannot and should not trust at all? If you answered yes to any of these questions, you are probably thinking of trust in all-or-nothing terms. Perhaps you feel you must trust completely or never trust anyone, and you feel forced to choose one of these two extremes. There is, however, a large gray area.

Trust is not all or nothing, rather it is a specific judgment about relying on someone for something you need in a specific situation. The meaning and degree of trust can change if any of these elements changes. As we said earlier in this chapter, trust can vary depending on a number of factors. Exercise 5.1 (see pages 154–155) asks you to consider how your degree of trust in yourself and other people changes in various situations. Complete that exercise now. Each line describes a specific area of basic human need that requires some measure of trust in yourself and in others. Your answers should give you a sense of how your decision to trust changes or doesn't change across situations.

How much you trust or don't trust in a specific situation is not important by itself. What matters most is whether the amount of trust matches the real situation. You may have excellent reasons for not trusting a *particular* person, but that is not good evidence for concluding that *no one* can be trusted. People are different. People are also imperfect. When a trusted person lets you down, does that mean they can never be trusted again? What evidence do you use for deciding how much to trust yourself or another? In Exercise 5.2 (see pages 156–157), we ask you to consider what evidence you have for making a particular judgment. Take a look at Exercise 5.1, in which you rated how much you trust in a specific situation. Pick an item or situation that you rated as most trusting by circling 1 or 2; then pick a situation in which you were least trusting (5 or 6). What evidence supports your belief that it is safe or not safe to trust in that situation?

As we said before, a decision to trust comes out of weighing four considerations. We have listed those again for you in Box 5.1 (see page 158). The first two factors affect how much weight you give to the evidence; the last two considerations are the evidence—your own past experiences and the particulars of the situation. Consider your specific situation in light of these four factors. Ask yourself, how strong was your need to trust in that situation? What was the risk in trusting? What past experiences with trust guided your decision? What other information did you have about the per-

EXERCISE 5.1 Rating How Much You Trust

Circle the number for how trustworthy you think yourself and others are in each of the following situations. When answering, think of recent situations from your day-to-day life. *Do not use a traumatic situation for this or any exercise.*

Circle

1. Extremely trustworthy	4. Slightly untrustworthy
2. Moderately trustworthy	5. Moderately untrustworthy
3. Slightly trustworthy	6. Extremely untrustworthy

How much do you trust yourself	Extremely trustworthy				Extremely untrustworthy	
to listen to your feelings	1	2	3	4	5	6
to know what you like	1	2	3	4	5	6
to know what you dislike	1	2	3	4	5	6
to follow your instincts	1	2	3	4	5	6
to make decisions	1	2	3	4	5	6
to solve your own problems	1	2	3	4	5	6
to know *when* to trust	1	2	3	4	5	6
to know *how much* to trust	1	2	3	4	5	6
to know whom to trust	1	2	3	4	5	6
A family member						
to provide practical help (e.g., help moving, babysitting)	1	2	3	4	5	6
to offer support when I have a personal problem	1	2	3	4	5	6
to provide emotional comfort	1	2	3	4	5	6

EXERCISE 5.1   (continued)

Circle

1. Extremely trustworthy	4. Slightly untrustworthy
2. Moderately trustworthy	5. Moderately untrustworthy
3. Slightly trustworthy	6. Extremely untrustworthy

	Extremely trustworthy				Extremely untrustworthy	
A friend						
to provide practical help	1	2	3	4	5	6
to provide support when I have a personal problem	1	2	3	4	5	6
to provide emotional comfort	1	2	3	4	5	6
A neighbor						
to provide practical help	1	2	3	4	5	6
to provide support when I have a personal problem	1	2	3	4	5	6
to provide emotional comfort	1	2	3	4	5	6
A stranger						
to provide practical support (i.e., give directions, help carry a heavy bag out to the car from the store)	1	2	3	4	5	6

EXERCISE 5.2 Weighing the Evidence on How Safe It Is to Trust

How much do you trust yourself and others in specific circumstances? Next to (A) below, list a circumstance from Exercise 5.1 in which you judged yourself as *most trustworthy* (1or 2). Next to (B) below, list a situation in which you judged yourself as *most untrustworthy* (5 or 6). Then list all the facts or evidence you have both for and against the accuracy of the rating.

A. Pick a situation from Exercise 5.1 in which you rated yourself as most trustworthy. Write it here:

____

____

What facts or evidence support this rating as accurate?

a. ____________________________________

b. ____________________________________

c. ____________________________________

What facts or evidence indicate this rating is not accurate?

a. ____________________________________

b. ____________________________________

c. ____________________________________

B. What situation did you rate yourself as most *un*trustworthy (5 or 6)?

____

____

What evidence (facts) supports this belief as accurate?

a. ____________________________________

b. ____________________________________

c. ____________________________________

What evidence (facts) supports this belief as not accurate?

a. ____________________________________

b. ____________________________________

c. ____________________________________

EXERCISE 5.2 (continued)

Next to (C) below, list a circumstance from Exercise 5.1 in which you judged another person as *most trustworthy* (1 or 2). Next to (D) below, list a situationn in which you judged another person as *most untrustworthy* (5 or 6). Then list all the facts or evidence you have both for and against the accuracy of the rating.

C.   Pick a situation from Exercise 5.1 in which you rated someone as most trustworthy and write it here:

_____

_____

What facts or evidence support this rating as accurate?

    a. _____

    b. _____

    c. _____

What facts or evidence indicate this rating is not accurate?

    a. _____

    b. _____

    c. _____

D.   What situation did you rate someone as most untrustworthy (5 or 6)?

_____

_____

What evidence (facts) supports this belief as accurate?

    a. _____

    b. _____

    c. _____

What evidence (facts) support this belief as not accurate?

    a. _____

    b. _____

    c. _____

son and the situation? When you finish, move on to the next section to consider what your answers mean.

BOX 5.1   Factors to Weigh When Deciding Whether to Trust

- The degree of your need
- The degree of risk
- Your past experiences with trust
- Any other information you have about the particular person and situation

---

DO YOU FEEL TRUSTING ENOUGH?

Are you getting your basic needs for trust met? Everyone needs to be able to trust self and others at some basic level. How do you respond to the following statements?

I generally trust my ability to make decisions.	___ yes	___ no
I rely on my gut feelings to know what I like and dislike.	___ yes	___ no
I have friends I can depend on.	___ yes	___ no

Did you answer "no" to any of these questions? If so, your capacity to trust may be constricted or disrupted. If you trust others but not your own feelings or judgment, you may trust when it is not safe to do so. If you trust yourself but don't depend on others, you may be struggling in your relationships. It is a huge and unnecessary burden to rely only on yourself. It is exhausting, lonely, and ultimately not enough. We need other people. We need to trust ourselves and others. Despite the emotional risk, we sometimes must depend on others. If you think you could have a problem with trust, continue reading. The next section helps you begin to track where you are in the area of trust.

TRACKING REACTIONS TO BELIEFS ABOUT TRUST

Identifying Your Beliefs about Trust

The exercises so far may have reminded you of at least one particular situation, since the trauma, in which you felt a problem with trust. Perhaps someone let you down, or you wanted to ask for help but couldn't quite trust anyone enough to ask. Perhaps you don't trust yourself in some way. Think of that situation and then use it to complete Exercise 5.3 (see page 160).

Bonnie completed Exercise 5.3 to identify what beliefs she might have about trust. After a terrible accident, she had joined a support group of survivors. She wanted help, but once in the group she found it very difficult to talk. She felt guarded even though the other group members encouraged her to share. She was thinking of that situation when she came to the first space in the exercise. For "Situation" she wrote

I don't trust myself to talk about my feelings in the group.

Following the instructions, Bonnie then looked at what she had just written and asked herself, "What does this say about me?" She next wrote

If I talk about my feelings, I'm afraid I will cry.

Bonnie then asked herself what that said about her.

It's weak to cry. If I cry, I'll feel ashamed afterward and want to close myself off even more from other people.

Bonnie then thought about what this said about her. After thinking for awhile she wrote

It's not so much being afraid of the group, as being afraid of the aftermath inside me. I am afraid that if I cry, it will take a long time for me to get back to normal. I'll feel terrible about myself because if I cry that says I'm a weak person.

The last question in the exercise asked Bonnie to consider all that she had written down so far in the exercise. Can she draw any conclusions about herself from these statements? She wrote

I don't trust myself to control my feelings in the group.

❧ EXERCISE 5.3   Identifying Beliefs about Trust

Do not use a traumatic situation for this exercise. Think instead of a recent situation in which you think you had a problem trusting either yourself or another person. If you cannot think of such a situation, consider a situation you judged as untrustworthy in Exercise 5.1. Do you wish your answer could be different? Describe the situation in the first space below, then write what you think that situation says about you. What does it mean about you that you judged the situation as untrustworthy? After you write a response, look at what you wrote. Then write what that says about you. Continue answering the questions by looking at your immediately preceding answer.

Situation:

_____

_____

What does this say or mean about me?

_____

_____

Looking at what I just wrote, what does *that* say or mean about me?

_____

_____

What does *that,* in turn say or mean about me?

_____

_____

Looking at all the above, can I drawn any conclusions about me?

_____

_____

Adapted with permission from Dennis Greenberger and Christine Padesky, *Mind Over Mood: Change How You Feel by Changing the Way You Think.* New York: Guilford Press, 1995.

Bonnie wants to be strong. If she talks about her feelings, however, she is afraid that she will cry, even though she tries not to. She believes that this means she is weak. How can she trust herself to be strong when it comes to feelings? She thinks she can't. Bonnie's belief about trust is also connected to issues of control. (She might find it helpful to read Chapter 6 on power and control also.) In the meantime, her belief seems to be interfering with her need to trust herself as well as other people. Clearly the belief seems to have drawbacks, but it probably also has advantages.

Evaluating How a Belief Helps and Hinders You

Exercise 5.4 (see page 162) asks you to consider both the advantages and the drawbacks of any beliefs you have identified. Every belief will have some of each, but the overall balance may lean more toward helping you or hindering you. We will look at how Bonnie did with this exercise in the next section.

Bonnie started Exercise 5.4 by writing down her conclusion from the last line of the previous exercise. She wrote:

I don't trust myself to control my feelings.

Then she started circling the numbers for how much the belief helped or hindered her in the group. When she thought about it, she felt that the belief was helpful in the group. It helped her stay in control, although it was not helping her connect or rely on the other group members. There was no middle number to circle, so she just skipped that question for now. The next question asked how calming or upsetting was the belief. She thought it had a calming effect. Without the belief holding her back, she thought she'd be crying and that would make her pretty upset. On the other hand, it seemed kind of inflexible, although it did help her feel safer. She thought the belief helped her understand herself and feel good about herself as a strong person—as long as she could stay strong. But that was the problem—it was so hard to hold back. She wasn't sure she could keep up the strong facade. It did tend to make her feel hopeless. How was she ever going to connect and get the support she needed? How could she get support without feeling she was a terrible, out-of-control weakling? When she thought about how essential the belief was to survival, she realized that it wasn't exactly a life-or-death issue. On the other hand, when she thought about losing control of her feelings, crying, and being a weak person, she felt a sense of great danger. She

EXERCISE 5.4   How Does This Belief Help and Hinder Me?

Most beliefs have both advantages and disadvantages. Consider those for the belief you identified in the last line of Exercise 5.3. Write down the belief in the space below, then circle how helpful or hindering the belief is for each question.

Belief: _____

Circle

1. Extremely helpful	4. Not at all helpful
2. Very helpful	5. Gets in my way
3. Moderately helpful	6. Gets in my way a lot

	Extremely helpful				**Gets in my way a lot**	
1. How helpful is this belief?	1	2	3	4	5	6
2. How calming is this belief?	1	2	3	4	5	6
3. How flexible is this belief?	1	2	3	4	5	6
4. How safe does this belief make me feel?	1	2	3	4	5	6
5. Does this belief help me understand myself?	1	2	3	4	5	6
6. Does this belief give me hope?	1	2	3	4	5	6
7. How essential is the belief to my survival?	1	2	3	4	5	6
8. How well does this belief help me cope?	1	2	3	4	5	6
9. Does the belief help me make sense of the world?	1	2	3	4	5	6
10. Does this belief help me make decisions?	1	2	3	4	5	6
11. Does this belief help me know what I need for myself?	1	2	3	4	5	6

decided that it was important to her survival to be strong. She circled 3, moderately essential for her survival.

When Bonnie considered the question of whether the belief helped her cope, she felt it had to be a 1, extremely helpful in helping her cope. Bonnie understood coping as being able to not cry, to stay composed, in control, not get emotional. On the other hand, being this way could be very difficult. If coping was all about making a hardship easier to bear, then being strong and not crying didn't really feel all that much easier. The easy way was to cry, to let herself fall to pieces. That's why not crying meant she was strong—*because* it was a difficult thing to do. This sense of strength was partly how she made sense of the world; it helped guide her decisions. It helped her know what she needed for herself. She needed to be strong. When Bonnie finished marking her answers, she looked at the whole exercise. Overall, she had marked the belief as having more benefits than drawbacks.

If the advantages of a belief outweigh its disadvantages for you, you may not need to complete the rest of the exercises in the chapter. You may choose to start with another chapter in this workbook. However, if you feel you do not have as much trust as you would like in your life, you may want to identify other beliefs about trust and weigh their pros and cons. People usually have more than just one belief about trust. Bonnie wasn't sure if the belief she had identified really was a problem or not as it seemed to have more advantages than disadvantages. On the other hand, she felt she wasn't as trusting as she'd like to be. She thought she'd go a little further in the chapter with this belief to see what else might come up.

Pinpointing Problem Areas to Think Through Further

If you have a problem with trust, is it a problem trusting yourself or a problem trusting others? If you think you have problems in both areas, start first by working on trust in yourself.

Look back now at how you completed Exercise 5.1. If your problem is with trusting yourself, look at the first section of that exercise. Review the nine ways you might or might not trust yourself. Is the belief you identified similar to any of these ways of trusting yourself? As we said earlier, each of the items requires some measure of trust, either in yourself or in others. If your problem is trusting others, look at the remainder of Exercise 5.1. Does the problem with other people concern relying on them for practical help? or emotional support and comfort?

Bonnie wasn't sure she had a problem with trust, but if she did, it seemed to be about trusting herself. She looked at the items in the first part of Exercise 5.1 with her belief, "I don't trust myself to control my feelings," in mind. The phrase "to listen to your feelings" was there at the top. That was very close to her belief. A bit later in the list there was also the phrase "to follow your instincts." Sometimes instincts are called "gut feelings." She had not thought much about these items when she initially filled out this exercise but now it struck her as odd that the items were there at all. The exercise was saying that people need to be able to trust their feelings and instincts. But in Bonnie's view, feelings and instincts were not to be trusted at all. That's why they needed to be controlled. These items in the list seemed to contradict her belief that feelings need to be controlled. Control, however, is as much a basic human need as is trust. Does Bonnie have to choose between trusting herself and controlling herself? The more she thought about her answers to the exercises, the more she realized that this was exactly how she saw the situation.

If any of the items in Exercise 5.1 don't make sense to you, or if they contradict what you think trust means, that is important information. If one of the five basic needs seems to cancel out or prevent you from getting other needs met, you are likely thinking in all-or-nothing terms. Bonnie only now realized that she was indeed thinking that feelings could not be trusted *at all* and that they had to be *completely* controlled. She was beginning to wonder if trusting her feelings could somehow coexist with controlling her feelings. What might that look like? What might trust and control mean if she is to have them both? Beginning to identify and explore her beliefs was the first important step in the process for Bonnie to ultimately find ways to get her needs met.

Taking Stock

Pause now to consider what you need and want. If you wish, you can put this work aside for now. Do you need to take care of yourself now and find comfort? Feel free to do so. If you prefer to move on to other chapters and issues in this workbook, feel free to do that. Do you want to continue working on issues related to trust? Exercise 5.5 asks you to take stock of where you are now in working on trust. Fill this out as a record, then move on with whatever you need to do right now.

EXERCISE 5.5   Taking Stock of Your Work on Trust

Consider what you think and feel right now. Do you wish take a break from this work? Do you wish to continue? Please check the statements that describe your situation right now.

_____ 1. My beliefs about trusting myself are fine. I do not need to think them through further. I feel as trustworthy as I need to feel.

_____ 2. My beliefs about trusting others are fine. I do not need to think them through further. I feel as trusting of others as I need to feel.

_____ 3. There are ways that I might not be as trusting of myself as I could be, but I don't want to think further about this right now. I can come back to work on this chapter when I feel ready.

_____ 4. There are ways that I might not be as trusting of others as I could be, but I don't want to think further about this right now. I can come back to work on this chapter when I feel ready.

_____ 5. I am beginning to think about why some of my beliefs about trust do not work. I can continue working on this, but I want to move slowly and carefully and can stop this work at any time.

_____ 6. I am ready to think through my beliefs about trust.

If you checked 5 or 6 above, write down here any beliefs that you may wish to work on further now or at some future time:

_____

_____

_____

_____

_____

_____

_____

_____

_____

THINKING THROUGH BELIEFS ABOUT TRUST

The exercises in the rest of this chapter help you look more closely at beliefs you may have about trust. Remember to take care of yourself as you do these exercises. Do you remember your self care plan for triggers (p. 16)? Review the plan you completed in the prologue. Stop if memories or emotions of the trauma are triggered. Stop and do one of these activities if you feel you may become emotionally overwhelmed.

Choosing Beliefs to Work On

Make a list of the beliefs you have identified so far. Perhaps you have none, only one, or several. Write down any that you have below:

_____

_____

_____

Now consider which of the beliefs you would like to think through more completely. For each belief, think it through by filling out Exercise 5.6 (see pages 168–169). As we saw in Chapter 4, you can start by reusing the same situation you used to identify the belief; or you can choose another situation that may fit better.

Let's look at how Bonnie thought through the belief "I don't trust my self to control my feelings."

Sort Out the Facts of What Happened

The first question in Exercise 5.6 asked Bonnie to describe the facts of a particular situation. She used the example of the group again. She wrote

The people in the group talk about how they feel, and they encourage me to talk about how I feel. Once I did start to talk about the accident and my feelings, but I lost control and started to cry.

Sort Out the Meaning the Facts Have for You

The next question asked how Bonnie interpreted this situation. She had already answered this, in a way, in the earlier exercise, but she described it again.

> Talking about my feelings makes me lose control. I cry, then I feel ashamed and terrible about myself for being weak.

Identify the Underlying Belief

Bonnie took the meaning one step further to state the lesson she saw in this meaning and experience.

> It's weak to cry. It's weak to lose control of your feelings.

The next question asked when she first started to believe this. This was hard to answer because it seemed as if she had known forever that it was weak and shameful to cry. It must have gone back into childhood. Big girls don't cry. Only sissies cry. Being strong and tough meant you could take whatever got dished out without complaining. Being strong means being able to handle things on your own.

Evaluate the Pros and Cons of the Belief

Bonnie then thought about how this statement made her think and feel about herself. Crying made her feel ashamed and terrible. When she felt in control and composed, she felt better about herself. Still, it was difficult to keep herself together. That's why she'd joined the support group, because it felt so bad toughing it out by herself. She wished she could let down her guard and count on group members to help her—but that would mean admitting she was weak and couldn't handle it on her own.

Bonnie thought about how this belief helped and protected her. She looked back at her answers to Exercise 5.4. The belief helped keep her from crying and so it helped keep her from feeling weak, ashamed, and terrible about herself. On the other hand, it was holding her back in the group and in other relationships. It was a burden to feel she had to be strong all the time, to stay in control.

EXERCISE 5.6   Steps for Thinking Through a Belief about Trust of Self or Others

The belief you wish to think through:

_____

Sort Out the Facts of What Happened

Think of a particular situation in which this belief may have been a problem. You can use the same situation you used to identify the belief, or use another situation in which trust was an issue. Describe the facts. What happened? What was the sequence of events?

Sort Out the Meaning the Facts Have for You

How did you interpret this situation? What did it mean to you?

Identify the Underlying Belief

What lesson did you draw from it about yourself? About other people?

When did you start believing this about yourself or others? Was this incident the first time? If not, when and how do you remember first learning this lesson?

Evaluate the Pros and Cons of the Belief

How does believing this make you feel about yourself or others? What does it make you think about yourself or others?

How does believing this help you or protect you?

How does believing this hold you back or get in your way?

Imagine Alternative Meanings for the Same Facts

Look back at your description of what happened (the first question above). Are there other ways to interpret what happened? What else could the situation mean? Is there an alternative meaning that would fit the facts of what happened? If so, what is it?

Evaluate the Pros and Cons of the Alternative Meaning

What positive feelings do you have when you think about this alternative meaning?

What negative feelings do you have when you think about this alternative meaning?

Consider How to Check the Accuracy of These Beliefs

How could you test to see whether or not your belief is true?

How high is the risk if you test the truth of what you believe? How dangerous would it be?

What good things might happen if you test the truth of what you believe?

Put the Process in Perspective

Will testing the belief matter 10 years from now? Would it help or hinder you in the future?

Imagine Alternative Meanings for the Same Facts

This question asked Bonnie to look back at her description of the facts. The facts were that she had lost control and cried when she talked about her feelings. Could this mean something else other than that she was a weak person? What else could it mean? It seemed almost impossible that this could mean something else. Then she remembered an earlier exercise in the chapter. It had raised the possibility that feelings could sometimes be trusted and if so, they might not always need to be controlled. If that were the case, then crying might sometimes not be so terrible. Could it ever be a good thing to cry? If it could be good, maybe that meant she wasn't so weak?

Evaluate the Pros and Cons of the Alternative Meaning

As Bonnie thought about the possibility that it could be a good thing to cry, she just couldn't quite believe how it might be real. However, she noticed a little glimmer of relief that flashed through her mind as she wondered if it could ever be a good thing to cry. This also scared her. It felt as though she could easily cry when she thought of the alternative meaning and that made her feel frightened of losing control.

When Bonnie thought of the worst thing that could happen, she thought about falling to pieces, crying and not being able to stop, being totally out of control and humiliated. She imagined other people thinking less of her as she wallowed helpless and feeling sorry for herself.

Consider How to Check the Accuracy of the Belief

The only thing Bonnie could think of was letting herself cry again in the group. But why would this be any different from the time before? She didn't want to do that until she had some hope that it could be different. Then it occurred to her that maybe she could just ask the people in the group if they believed, as she did, that crying was weak. She wouldn't have to actually cry. She could tell them how she felt about it and see if they agreed or not. This seemed less of a risk.

But it was still difficult to imagine good things happening if she checked out the alternative belief. What would the other group members think? Would they care? Would it change things?

Put the Process in Perspective

Checking out her belief seemed a risky thing to do. But the next question asked how might she feel about it years from now. If she checked it out, and discovered everybody else agreed that she was a weak and terrible person, it would be humiliating, awful. In 10 years, however, it probably wouldn't make much of a difference. On the other hand, if it turned out that it could ever be all right to cry, then checking out the possibility could make a real difference over the long term.

This exercise asked Bonnie questions she had never thought to ask before. She still hadn't changed her mind about anything. She still felt she was correct in believing that

> I can't trust my feelings. Feelings need to be controlled. I'm weak if I lose control of my feelings and cry.

But she was surprised she was able to imagine an alternative meaning. She didn't believe there was much truth to it, but just being able to think of it was a good sign. As we mentioned earlier, flexibility is one of the 10 most effective ways of coping. It takes some flexibility just to be able to come up with alternative meanings and interpretations. Bonnie's alternative meaning was

> Maybe sometimes it can be a good thing to trust my feelings. Maybe crying doesn't mean I'm weak. Maybe sometimes it's normal.

Whenever she feels ready, Bonnie's next step is to collect evidence on the accuracy of what she believes as well as on the alternative interpretation. Bonnie felt she wasn't ready to do that yet. Instead, she decided to go on to the next chapter and look at issues of power and control. Later on, however, she did come back and pick up her work on trust.

Putting aside work in a need area and coming back to it later can be useful. When Bonnie came back and reviewed her answers to the exercises in this trust chapter, she saw things she hadn't seen before, for example, that trusting others meant she must give up trusting herself. It was only after Bonnie worked through Chapter 6 on control and power and Chapter 7 on self-esteem that these other aspects of trust became visible to her. Bonnie did eventually feel ready to check her beliefs against the evidence. Let's see how she did that.

WEIGHING THE EVIDENCE ON BELIEFS ABOUT TRUST

Weigh the Evidence on the Existing Belief

When Bonnie returned to her work on trust, before she did anything, she first had to *think* and *plan* carefully about how she might check her beliefs. Collecting evidence about her belief did *not* mean that she had to let go and cry in the group just to see what would happen. To her, this was a high-risk thing to do. It was, however, the first thing that came to her mind. It took some thinking before she could come up with lower risk ideas for collecting evidence.

Brainstorm Ideas for Collecting Evidence

Before you check the accuracy of your beliefs, you must come up with lots of ideas for how to do it without taking big risks. One way to gather ideas is to brainstorm. You can use Exercise 5.7 or use a blank piece of paper. Write down *all* the ideas that come into your head no matter how frightening, impractical, or silly you might think they are. Be prepared for the likelihood that the first ideas will be high risk; those are the ideas in the front of your mind. We do not want you to do anything high risk, but you can get those ideas out of the way by writing them down. This can make it easier for you then to come up with *low-risk* ideas. Write down whatever you can think of in whatever order you think of it. Be sure to brainstorm ideas for checking the alternative belief as well as for the old belief. Some ideas will work for both, but some may not.

To help you focus on low-risk ways to check your beliefs, remember that there are categories of low-risk evidence checking that may help you. These are the "baby steps" for testing a belief mentioned in Chapters 3 and 4. We want to review them again now. As you read them, think of your particular belief, and the alternative meaning. Think also of the situations you already find yourself in. Use the following list of baby steps to continue brainstorming. Make a list of whatever ideas pop into your head.

1. Notice or observe events or actions and the people acting.
2. Watch other people's reactions to the event or action.
3. Notice when you yourself are already carrying out actions that produce evidence about your belief.

**EXERCISE 5.7   Brainstorm Ideas for Collecting Evidence
on a Belief**

Create a list of rough ideas for collecting evidence on a belief. The goal is to come up with some low-risk ways to collect evidence, but be prepared that the first ideas you have may be high risk. Write them down to get them out of the way. You do not need to carry out *any* of the ideas you write down. You will screen these ideas later and discard any you choose. Begin by writing down a belief and an alternative interpretation on which you want to collect evidence. In the blank space below write down any and all ideas that come to you mind for how to do this.

Belief: _____

Alternative interpretation: _____

4. Ask friends questions about their reactions.

5. When it feels safe enough, take a small action with a safe friend and see how the friend reacts to you.

The lowest risk ways to test a belief usually consist of observing what is already going on around you. However, if you are to give the belief a fair and honest test, you need to plan in advance to watch for one thing in particular. Brainstorming low-risk ideas involves thinking about what specific actions or events to watch for. For example, Bonnie distrusted her feelings and believed that it was weak to cry. Therefore, she wanted to pay particular attention to anyone who cried or got teary in the group. She also wanted to pay attention to how the other group members reacted when someone cried. Trying to pay attention to both of these things at the same time is tempting, but it will divide Bonnie's attention and she could miss something important. If her plan is to work, she needs to focus on only one observation at a time. Observing how another person cries, and observing how others react to the crying person count as two different ways to collect evidence. Each time you can identify something specific to watch for, that one thing is its own separate idea.

Rank Ideas by Lowest Risk First

When you have brainstormed a number of specific ways you could collect evidence, the next step is to rank them according to risk. You can do this using the blank form in Exercise 5.8. In the spaces at the top of the form, write down your existing belief, and an alternative interpretation. Then, on your rough brainstorming list, review all the ideas you have written down and find the one with the lowest risk. Remember, you do *not* have to carry out *any* of the ideas you've written down. But if you did decide to try one, what would be the consequences? For which ideas are the worst consequences not that bad? Which idea seems the easiest and the safest to carry out? If you don't have any easy and safe ideas, you need to go back and do more brainstorming. Otherwise, write down the lowest risk idea at the top of the baby steps list directly under "Least Feared Actions/Observations." Then cross that idea off your rough list. Out of the remaining ideas on your rough brainstorming list, find the one that is now lowest risk. Write that on the second line of the baby steps list and cross it off your rough brainstorming

EXERCISE 5.8   Baby Steps for Testing a Belief about Trust

In the first blanks below, write down the belief you are thinking of testing and an alternative interpretation. When you have brainstormed ideas for possible ways to collect evidence on a belief, rank those ideas by risk, starting with the lowest risk ways. List only ways that are within a reasonable risk. *Do not list any high-risk ways to collect evidence.*

Belief: _____

Alternative interpretation: _____

Least Feared Actions/Observations

_____

_____

_____

_____

_____

_____

_____

_____

_____

_____

Most Feared Actions/Observations

list. Continue selecting the lowest risk idea from among those you have not yet crossed off the brainstorming list. At some point, you may find that the only ideas left have bad consequences. These ideas are not baby steps. High-risk ways to collect evidence do not belong on the baby steps list. You don't have to fill the list. If you have enough low-risk ideas to fill all 10 lines for baby steps, rank only the low- to reasonable-risk ideas you can safely imagine yourself doing.

Carry Out Lowest Risk Ways to Collect Evidence

Many of the lowest risk ways to collect evidence on a belief involve observation. Carrying this out can be trickier than you think. We tend to notice the facts that support our beliefs and miss those that do not. For this reason, you need to test an existing belief and an alternative interpretation together, at the same time. Do the facts you notice apply to both beliefs or only one and not the other? In collecting observations as evidence, you need to pay attention to the facts of what actually happens. This means being able to sort out the facts from your thoughts and feelings about it. For example, in the past someone in Bonnie's group did cry, but Bonnie felt the other's situation was very different from her own and so she dismissed the incident as having nothing to do with her. If she keeps doing that, her plan to collect evidence will not be very helpful to her. Bonnie needs to record the facts regardless of what she thinks or feels about them.

Record and Weigh the Evidence for and against the Belief

When you have created a list of small baby steps that can test the accuracy of your beliefs—both the existing one and the alternative one—you may be ready to start collecting the evidence. We enclose two sheets for recording evidence. Exercise 5.9 and Exercise 5.10 are basically the same except that one is for recording evidence of your existing belief and the other for evidence on the alternative meaning.

Bonnie made her list, and her first task was to observe anyone in her group who cried. During one group session, a man in the group began crying quietly as he talked about his experience. He seemed a little embarrassed afterward, but he didn't appear to be devastated over it. She realized that she herself did not see him as weak. Over the next few meetings, two other

EXERCISE 5.9 What Evidence Do I Have about the Existing Belief?

What evidence do you already have about the accuracy of your existing belief? What facts, words, or actions support the belief? What facts, words, or actions indicate the belief is inaccurate? Write those down below.

Belief: _____

What facts or evidence support this belief as accurate?

1. _____

2. _____

3. _____

What facts or evidence indicate this belief is not accurate?

1. _____

2. _____

3. _____

How sure are you that this belief is accurate? Mark how sure on the following scale. Use the second evaluation scale later to check on changes in your beliefs in light of new evidence.

Date: _____

Accurate   Inaccurate

_____

100%   50%   0%

Date: _____

Accurate   Inaccurate

_____

100%   50%   0%

❧ **EXERCISE 5.10   What Evidence Do I Have
                   about the Alternative Meaning?**

What evidence do you already have about the accuracy of the alternative meaning?
What facts, words, or actions support the alternative meaning? What facts, words, or
actions indicate the alternative meaning is inaccurate? Write those down below.

Alternative meaning: _____

What facts or evidence support this interpretation as accurate?

1. _____
2. _____
3. _____

What facts or evidence indicate this interpretation is not accurate?

1. _____
2. _____
3. _____

How sure are you that this interpretation is accurate? Mark how sure on the following
scale. Use the second evaluation scale later to check on changes in your beliefs in light
of new evidence.

Date: _____

Accurate   Inaccurate

_____

100%   50%   0%

Date: _____

Accurate   Inaccurate

_____

100%   50%   0%

women cried as they told their stories. These women didn't seemed to be embarrassed at all over crying. She also noticed that the other group members responded by looking sympathetic, listening quietly, and saying supportive things afterward. Bonnie thought about her observations carefully and decided that she could, at least, try to tell the group how difficult it was for her to talk. She thought she could do this without actually crying. Briefly in one session she mentioned how awful she felt about herself when she cried. Other group members told her they didn't see crying that way at all. One of the women who cried earlier said it helped her and that she felt better afterward, not worse. Others said they didn't think crying was a sign of weakness. Moving slowly at her own pace, Bonnie felt safe enough in the group to tell her story, even though she realized she would cry—and she did cry as she told her whole story. The group members comforted her afterward, and she couldn't believe how relieved she felt after crying. She slept better that night than she had in all the weeks since the accident.

Keeping your attention on the evidence with an open mind over time will help you find your way once again. It will not happen overnight, but we have seen it happen in good time.

SUMMARIZING YOUR WORK ON TRUST

Consider now what you need for yourself. You can put this workbook aside for now, or you can continue to work on it as you choose. You may move on to the next chapter in the workbook or you can revisit parts of this chapter on trust or earlier chapters. Feel free to identify other beliefs about trust, evaluate them, and test how accurate they may be. When you are ready to stop your work on trust for the time being, complete Exercise 5.11 as a summary of your work. You can return to issues of trust at any time. Reviewing this summary when you come back will give you a sense of where you are and what else you might want to work on.

Trust is a basic need, but it does not have to be total. Trust can be partial and vary according to your own need and the risk. The path back to trust is based on an honest acknowledgment of the risk, together with an honest acknowledgment of the evidence. There is no trust without some measure of risk, but that risk does not have to be extreme or unreasonable. It can be based on evidence that the person or thing has proved worthy of that trust.

EXERCISE 5.11   Summarizing Your Work on Trust

I have identified the following beliefs about trust:

I can think of the following alternative meanings:

I have already carried out the following steps (mark with X); or I would like in the future to carry out the following steps (mark with *):

_____ Make a list of what evidence might confirm and/or contradict the existing belief.

_____ Organize the list of evidence from least feared/least risky to collect to most feared/most risky to collect.

_____ Carry out the least feared/least risky way to collect evidence.

_____ Keep a record of the evidence collected—both pro and con.

List here any evidence collected—what did you see or do, and how did it turn out? Continue adding to this list over time, as you become aware of additional evidence.

As you end this chapter, remember how it feels to trust yourself and to have that trust rewarded. Remember how it feels to trust another person, to rely on another for something you need, and to have that person come through for you. If you know how trust feels, you can come safely to feel it again.

CHAPTER SIX

REGAINING CONTROL IN YOUR LIFE

YOUR NEED FOR POWER AND CONTROL: The need to feel in charge of your own actions; the need to have some influence or impact on others.

WHAT THE WEAK DON'T KNOW about the process of the power relationship is their own strength.

—Elizabeth Janeway, *Powers of the Weak*

HOW CONTROL AND POWER CAN BE ISSUES AFTER TRAUMA

We all need some sense of self-control and personal power, based on the ability to control ourselves, to have an effect on other people, and an effect on our environment. Trauma, however, is often an experience of being overpowered by outside forces. It can involve the forceful invasion of your environment on your body. Floods, bombs, hurricanes, fires, or earthquakes are powerful events that overwhelm efforts to control them. Sometimes the overpowering outside force is another person such as a rapist, burglar, abusive family member, or battering spouse. During your trauma experience, your only option may have been to submit or you may have fought, struggled and still been overpowered. You may have had to stand by helplessly while another was harmed. Whatever happened, you may know first-hand how it feels to be overpowered, helpless, and out-of-control. You may continue to feel helpless, even after the trauma is over. You can recover a sense of power, but you may not realize that your trauma reactions have anything to do with this issue. If any of the following descriptions resemble your experience, you could be helped by reading further in this chapter.

Loss of Self-Control

After trauma you may feel less in control of your thoughts and emotions. The sudden intrusion of emotions is called *emotional flashbacks.*

❀ *Every time Meg thinks of her mother, she remembers the car crash that killed her. Then Meg feels an overwhelming wave of grief. She sees the crushed car and then can't stop the tears that pour out. Emotions flood her and she feels out of control. She wonders if she is going crazy.*

Meg's feelings are not unusual after trauma although not everyone feels this way—or if they do, it may be for only a short while. Some people are able to suppress the memory of what happened and the upsetting feelings that go with it.

❀ *Jim, a police officer, was involved in dead body identification in a major disaster. At first he was flooded by horrible images and overwhelming feelings, but he has tried to bury the feelings so that he could continue doing his job. He has been able to hold back the worst of it. As time goes on, however, he no longer feels much joy in his life. At times, he feels that he is not part of the real world. He feels numb, has become cynical, and says he cannot see beauty in the world around him.*

In different ways, Meg and Jim are both experiencing a disrupted sense of control in their emotional lives. You may sometimes feel as though you are going crazy and that, if others knew, they would think so too. You might fear that no one would understand; they might even blame you for what happened. You may fear that if you were to talk about your experience, you would become even more crazy and out of control. These thoughts silence many survivors. But emotional flashbacks, and/or feelings of numbness and unreality are *normal* reactions to *abnormal* events. Making sense of a traumatic experience helps the feeling of being crazy go away. The more you understand yourself and what has happened, the less you will think you are out of control.

Loss of Power to Affect the World and Other People

We need to feel that our emotions, actions, or mere presence can make a difference. It is natural to want some influence on the decisions and actions of others. Following trauma, some survivors lose any sense that they can affect people or things outside themselves. You may feel helpless, powerless. You may feel that nothing you do will change anything, that action is useless. Or you may want to prove that this isn't true and so try to control everything. You may never want to feel out of control again.

> ❊ *Dan had been a platoon leader in Vietnam. He felt responsible for the men who served under him, yet daily he saw them killed. When he returned home, he tried to regain the sense of control he felt before his combat experience. He tried to control family and coworkers. People were often irritated with him. They did not understand he was trying to be protective. Dan had to work hard to understand his feelings of responsibility and what that meant in combat versus in his civilian life.*

It is likely that you were unable to control what happened to you during your traumatic experience. The truth is you may have been completely powerless in one or more ways. That sense of powerlessness may remain. You may no longer feel able to solve problems or meet daily challenges in your life. The sense of power you had before may be gone. Still, there are sources of power that remain with you. If you can recognize them, you will begin to regain some sense of control in your life.

Trauma Survivors Speak about Control and Power

- To me, power means choice. Although I cannot always choose what will happen in my life, I alone have the power to choose how I will respond to my circumstances. This power of choice gives me control and enables me to act in my own best interest.
- Power is having control and taking charge.
- Power is the ability to affect a situation, to bring or assist in bringing about a positive result. It is the urge to overcome or change.
- Power has nothing to do with what is fair.
- Power comes from taking charge, being able to make decisions. I can't even order from a menu without having an anxiety attack.
- One person is weak and one person is strong. One person makes the rules and the other person follows them. One person gives at his pleasure and the other person can only wait and hope. Or one person takes what he wants and the other person has no choice.

WHAT CAN IT MEAN TO BE POWERFUL AND IN CONTROL?

Trauma can result from the abuse of power such as interpersonal violence, coercion, or other forms of force. Power can be used to force someone to do something he or she does not want to do. For these reasons, control and power can seem evil and frightening at the same time that they seem essential for protection. Experiencing misuse of power can be terrible. You may think that being powerful can mean only using force or threatening to use force, making others feel helpless, humiliated, or belittled. Perhaps you have come to feel that there are only two kinds of people: those with power and those without. You may think there is no middle ground and you must choose. For some people, having even a little power may feel frightening.

> ❧ *Lynn grew up in a home in which the women took care of the house and of the men in the family. As a girl, Lynn's own feelings and needs were disregarded. Without question, her father's and other male relatives' needs always came first. For these reasons, Lynn felt unable to tell anyone when her older brother began abusing her. She felt treated like a doormat, but whenever she tried to stand up for herself, she would quickly back down. Standing up for herself felt too much like being abusive and demanding herself.*

As she grew up, Lynn saw only two examples of power: being powerless and at risk for abuse, or being powerful and abusive. If these extremes are the only possible options, then it's reasonable to conclude that power must *always* be abusive. But are these the only options? All parents have power over their children but not all parents are abusive. What else might power and control mean?

Power is the ability to make something happen. There are two parts to this definition. The first is to be able to act; the second is to have an effect. *Any* human action that has an effect, including speech, contains power. This power is not, however, all or nothing. The measure of power in any action may be very small, very large, or somewhere in between. The amount of power, the ability to do something, exists along a continuum. A range in strength or degree is not the only way that power can vary.

Power also has variations in method. There are many different ways to make something happen. Power does not have to be destructive or coercive. A movie or song can be powerful because it moves us, stirring our emotions.

The muscles in your legs have the power to move the rest of your body across the room. Power and control can mean many different things depending on *what* is happening and *how*.

Power can be out of control, but control is never without some power. Control is a form of power. It is the ability to make happen what you *want* to happen. Control implies intention, the ability to direct energy to have a particular effect. We often think of control as an ability to restrain or direct what is happening completely but control does not have to be total to be effective. A dam controls a river by blocking it, stopping its flow. A light switch controls a lamp by blocking electricity or letting it flow to a light bulb. In these instances, however, the entire river is not completely controlled, nor is all electricity completely controlled. Control does not have to be complete to be powerful and effective, nor does it have to involve blocking or restraint, although it can. Control is very often the result of knowledge or skill as much as of force or restraint. The muscles in your hands have the power to shape a lump of clay. But raw power alone cannot make the clay into the shape of a horse or a face.

There is raw power in the wind but its degree and meaning depend on what is being affected. There is some power in wind ruffling dune grass but the effect is not large. However, the same wind can power a sailboat across water. A boat, the wind, or a sailor, by itself, do not have great power. But the power can increase dramatically when all three interact. Although power is sometimes thought of as a thing or possession, it can also be thought of as a process. The power in a racing sailboat comes out of the entire interaction of the boat, the wind, and the sailor. Power as a process can arise out of relationships. It can shift and change when any of the circumstances in a relationship change.

A sense of control can be gained, temporarily, through brute force and can be lost the same way. Most of the time, however, it is gained through knowledge plus the skill to act on that knowledge. Although this kind of control can be lost when a situation changes, it can also be more readily regained. For example, the sails of a boat can go slack when the wind shifts and power will be lost; but power can be regained if the sailor knows what adjustments to make. The sailor's effectiveness depends on how well she knows her ship and the winds. Her ability to make the boat move and control its motion is based on knowledge plus her skill in acting on that knowledge. A key part of the sailor's power comes from knowing what she can and can't control. When the wind shifts, the sailor may wish she could change the wind back, but she won't get anywhere if she tries. Being powerful means knowing where and where not to put your efforts.

The Sources and Limitations of Personal Power and Control

Your sense of being in control, of having personal power, begins with how well you know and accept yourself. The foundation of your power is not control but self-knowledge. How well do you know your thoughts and feelings, what you like and dislike? Do you have difficulty paying attention to these things in yourself? Do you think you shouldn't feel or think the way you really do? Do you have trouble accepting your emotions? Do you often try to change them?

Your honest feelings and thoughts are a source of personal power if you know them and know how to use (and not use) them. They are like the wind for a sailor; they can help direct and propel you. But trying to change how you really feel is like a sailor trying to change the way the wind is blowing. When you try to control things that are not really under your control, it can make you feel completely out of control.

Trying to control feelings and thoughts by force does not usually work well, and when it does, there is a very high price. Feelings and thoughts come from who we really are. Listening to our thoughts and feelings is how we learn about ourselves, what we want, what we don't want, what we care about, what is and isn't important to us. Trying to change those messages cuts us off from who we are and from knowing what we want. Remember, control is the power to make what you want happen. To lose touch with what you really want *is* to lose control. To be in touch with your deepest feelings and thoughts and to choose actions based on them is one definition of integrity. There is power in integrity. It has an effect on others because they admire and respect it, not because they fear it.

While you cannot always control what you feel and think, you can control what you do with that information. You can choose whether or not to express what you think and feel. You can choose how to express it. You have control over your own actions.

You cannot, however, control the actions of other people. In the end, people control their own individual actions, just as you control your own.

You can, of course, express what you want and hope that it influences others, but ultimately what people do is up to them. This does not mean you are powerless; you have great power in your own ability to act and express what you want.

Sometimes individuals or governments try to control others completely. Great incentives are given for people to choose to behave the way those in power want. People's choices can be drastically limited, and terrible punishments can be inflicted for "wrong" choices. This is what much abusive behavior is about. Such situations can occur where there is an extreme power imbalance. The balance is rarely all or nothing. There would be no need for punishments if the powerful were in complete and total control of others. As long as people have some basic choices, they retain some power to act or not act, to respond or not respond, to cooperate or not cooperate. However, the effect of such choices can be very small and the risks very high. In extreme circumstances, true choice—and with it power and responsibility—can temporarily shrink to nothing.

Power and responsibility are both connected to choice. When you have little or no choice in a situation, you have no power to affect what happens. Therefore, you are not responsible for what happens. Trauma can involve just such a situation. It is painful to acknowledge how little power we sometimes have during a crime, in an abusive situation, in an accident. It may seem better to go over and over what you might have done differently, trying to think of a way you might have controlled or prevented what happened. This can be helpful if you learn something useful for the future. Remember, however, that you did not have this knowledge going through the original event. We can only do the best we can in any given situation and most traumatic situations have elements of surprise, confusion, or coercion. They paralyze normal people with fear, catch them off-guard and frequently offer no way to resist or escape. You may come to realize there was nothing you could have done to change the situation. If you come to that place, offer yourself compassion and forgiveness. Let go of your sense of responsibility. When nothing you can do makes a difference, you bear no responsibility for what happens. A large part of healing from traumatic events involves forgiving yourself.

Having been powerless in the past does not mean you are powerless now. Being helpless, powerless, and out-of-control are products of a specific situation. When anything in that situation changes, the possibilities for power and control can change as well, although you may not see this at first. Regaining a sense of power and control involves recognizing there is a new situation, getting acquainted with it, gaining knowledge about it and yourself. You have probably changed as well.

Empowering Yourself

If you have been checking in with yourself as you read this book, you have been getting to know yourself better. If you have been engaging in self-care when you feel you need it, you have started empowering yourself. Perhaps you have learned to recognize and understand the important messages in your thoughts and feelings. Perhaps you are learning to have some control over your most difficult and overwhelming feelings. Empowerment starts with recognizing and respecting what you need and want. It grows as you learn skills for managing your emotions and begin to see choices for action. Each of the 10 basic coping strategies discussed in Chapter 2 is a tool for helping you sail the waters of your emotional life. Being able to comfort yourself when you need it, even if only in a small way, is an exercise of your personal power.

The exercise of personal power means choosing whether or not to act and if so, how. You have the power to say what you want. You can say no to what you don't want. You also have the power to say nothing. Silence can be as much a choice as speaking. If your traumatic experiences include physical or emotional abuse by another person, you probably learned to *not* express your feelings. To express them may have increased your risk of being harmed. You may also have learned that saying "no" did not work to protect you. In such circumstances, silence can be the only choice that makes sense. But is that the only choice you have now? Have your circumstances changed? If so, your range of choices has probably changed too.

We believe the ability to speak our feelings and needs is empowering even if you don't always get the reaction you want and even if you're not sure what it is you do want. Self-expression does not have to be high risk. If you have difficulty speaking, write letters to yourself or keep a journal to express your thoughts and feelings. Even if you are the only reader, writing can be a powerful means of self-expression.

When you can, trying to speak your feelings and wants out loud can help you know them better. For example, if you are unhappy with your boss but don't know what to do, you could talk about it to a close, trusted friend. Just hearing yourself talk may help you realize new things, see that there are choices and alternatives you had not seen before. Having more choices leads to a greater sense of control. Good things can escalate, building on each other. But first, you may need to break out of the opposite cycle where feeling out-of-control leads to silence, withdrawal, and further helplessness.

We do not always get what we want but we are less likely to get it if we don't speak about it or ever tell anyone. If you have been in a situation in which your voice was dismissed and ignored, you may have given up trying to say what you really feel or want. But the situation may have changed since then. You may have more personal power than you realize.

Having an Effect on Others

There is power in expressing *what* you feel and want but the degree of effectiveness, usually depends on *how* you express it. You may feel there are only two choices: to be silent and passive or to be demanding and aggressive. There is, however, a middle ground. It is to be assertive. Being assertive means stating your feelings and needs in a way that respects those of other people. There are two ways to be assertive: saying what you like, and saying what you don't like. It is important to know how to do both. For example, when you buy something, bring it home then find out it's damaged, do you have trouble taking it back to the store? If food you order in a restaurant comes cold or is unsatisfactory for some reason, would you send it back to the kitchen? If someone unfairly gets ahead of you in a line at a store counter, do you say anything to the person? Keeping quiet and not acting in these situations can increase your sense of powerlessness. Perhaps you believe your only other choice of action is to yell, lose your temper, and put the other person down. There are, however, other ways to act. You probably have more choices of action than you realize.

It is in your control to think before acting very angrily. It is in your control to calmly, kindly, yet firmly request that a problem be corrected. You may not be able to control your actions in this way right now. But it is in your power to learn. Such control is a skill that can be learned and practiced. For example, when you have disagreements, you can learn to negotiate with others. When you know how and where to look, it is often possible to find a solution that does not take away from either you or the other person. If you try, the needs of both people can often be met. If you wish to explore any of these issues further, an excellent resource is *Your Perfect Right: A Guide to Assertive Living*. It is listed in the recommended readings at the end of this workbook.

Boundaries

You have power over your own actions but not over the actions of others. Others have power over their own actions but not over yours. What happens at the boundaries between people? Having a clear sense of your own personal boundaries helps protect you from feeling victimized in your causal and close relationships. Boundaries are, in essence, your personal limits on what feels good, right, and comfortable to you with a particular person in a particular situation.

Boundaries are both physical and emotional. Only you can know your own boundaries and different people will have different boundaries. How much physical space do you need to feel comfortable talking with a stranger? If the stranger keeps shifting closer to you, at some point you will probably feel uncomfortable. When this happens, your boundary has been crossed. Perhaps you will take a step back to reestablish a more comfortable distance. Do you need more space to be comfortable talking with a stranger than with your sister? How much emotional information are you comfortable sharing with others? In intimate relationships, you will generally feel comfortable revealing fears, doubts, and worries. You may feel very uncomfortable revealing the same emotional information to a casual acquaintance, but you don't have to, nor do you have to end the relationship. Instead, you could continue to enjoy going to the movies with the acquaintance but not share stories you want to keep private. It is good to have a variety of boundaries.

Establishing and maintaining good boundaries takes several steps. First, it requires that you have a sense of where your boundaries are and how it feels when one has been crossed. The signal is usually a feeling of discomfort or unease. Second, you need to act to reestablish what does feel comfortable. Other people may not realize they've violated one of your boundaries. Only you know what your boundaries are and so you need to let others know.

A simple action such as taking a step back from the person you are speaking with may be all that's needed. Sometimes, you need to tell the other person what is making you uncomfortable and ask if he or she please wouldn't do that again. Sometimes this means telling the other person several times. You have the right and the power to end a relationship if the other person cannot respect your boundaries.

If your boundaries were violated either through verbal abuse or physical intrusion, it can be difficult to establish clear and appropriate boundaries in other relationships. You may be uncertain what your rights are, or even that comfortable boundaries can exist at all. If you do not have clear boundaries, you can become enmeshed in relationships with others. In other words, you could find it difficult to maintain a sense of control, and you may have trouble holding onto yourself as a separate, independently functioning adult. Knowing what is comfortable for you in different relationships, and how to keep to those limits, will help you feel safer and more in control in your relationships. In some situations, clearly enforcing your boundaries is very adaptive.

❋ *Trudy had learned from past experience that talking with her father left her feeling confused, frightened, and nauseated. When she responded to him passively or cordially, he contacted her more often and sometimes even stopped by her apartment to see her. She finally decided to no longer have contact with him. She told him this and asked him not to call or visit her. He did, however, still call her but when he did, she was firm and repeated the boundary she had set earlier. "I have asked you not to contact me. I am going to hang up now." Then she did exactly that. Before too long, he stopped calling.*

You can read more about these issues in *Boundaries and Relationships* or *Boundaries: Where You End and I Begin*. Both books are listed in the recommended readings in Appendix A.

Hurting Yourself

The power to act includes the power to injure yourself. Some trauma survivors find themselves doing this. Self-injury is a complicated subject we will not discuss in detail, but we want to mention it because of the important connection between self-injury, control, and feelings. The ways people harm themselves may include punching walls so hard there is severe bruising or broken bones. It can include abusing substances such as alcohol, illegal drugs, prescription drugs, inhalants, etc. It can include not eating, overeating, exercising to the point of pain, burning, or cutting yourself with a knife or some other sharp object. There are many complicated reasons survivors might deliberately hurt themselves. One person can have many reasons.

People who harm themselves often do so in a very private way. Their closest friends or family may not be aware it happens. They often feel a sense of shame that they harm themselves. They usually do not understand why they do it, and they often believe it is bizarre or crazy and so must be kept secret. Trauma survivors are especially vulnerable to harming themselves because trauma-related feelings can be so intense. This is particularly true if the trauma was violent and the person had no control. Survivors may not know how to express their feelings directly, or they may not want to. Harming themselves can become a way to "get the feelings out." Self-injury can be an expression of anger or rage. For individuals who feel very helpless in their lives and feel unable to have any control over what happens to them, self-injury can be an expression of personal power as if to say, "It's my body and this is one thing I do have a say about." One dilemma with this expression of personal power is that it too often repeats, in some form, something that was done to that person during a trauma.

> ❄ *When Kathy became very angry and frustrated with her family and the rest of the world, she drank heavily and used cocaine. At these times, she thought, "To hell with all of you." Then she felt powerful, fearless, and didn't care about anyone else. Eventually Kathy realized the drugs only numbed her feelings temporarily, as well as jeopardized her life. It was just like when she used to dissociate, or "numb out" when her uncle abused her years before.*

Kathy felt powerful using drugs, but it was a power turned against herself. The drugs actually reduced her ability to have the effect she wanted or to gain some control in her life. When she stopped using drugs, she missed the numbness but did not want to continue feeling victimized at her own hands. She wanted to experience a sense of power that lasted, and that she could draw on at any time. Kathy found such ways to feel powerful in relationships. She learned to hold her ground when she saw things differently from other people. She learned to express her feelings even in the presence of her family who didn't "do" feelings. If self-injury may be a problem for you, an excellent resource for both men and women is *Women Who Hurt Themselves* by Dusty Miller. You can find further information on this in the "General Trauma" section in the recommended readings.

WHAT DO POWER AND CONTROL MEAN TO YOU?

Personal Power and Self-Control

What does it mean for you to have "power"?

Power to do what?

Do you have any knowledge that might be a source of power for you? What is it?

Are you generally aware of your own feelings about yourself, other people, and the situations in which you find yourself?

Do you ever imagine yourself having great power and control? What would you make happen? How and why?

Do you feel in control of your own actions and behaviors? How do you exercise this control?

Do you think it is realistic to expect to have some control in some situations?

Have you ever experienced a sense of personal power? When? What were its sources?

How much control do you have over what happens in your future?

Do you believe society has assigned you power because you belong to a certain group (by gender, race, religion, ethnic background, education, income)?

Do you think you are at risk for being controlled by other people?

Have your sense of power and need for control changed since your trauma?

Do you ever express yourself through self-injury or self-destructive behavior? What do you do?

Does this behavior accomplish your goals?

How does this self-destructive behavior affect other people?

How does this self-destructive behavior affect you?

Understanding Your Physical Boundaries

Knowing your boundaries is important if you are to develop a sense of control in your relationships. One of the most important areas within your control is being touched. It is your right to decide who touches you, when, how, and where. You have the right to ask for touch or decline touch. Touch can be comforting and soothing when done in a safe, mutually agreed on way. Here are some questions to help you understand your physical boundaries.

If you think in terms of an arm's length, how much physical space (i.e., how many arm's lengths?) is most comfortable for you in the following kinds of relationships?

In an intimate relationship:

With a close friend:

With an acquaintance:

With a stranger:

Have you established rules for yourself about being touched? If so, what are they?

Can you think of a person with whom you have clear, comfortable boundaries? What do you and the other person do to maintain these boundaries?

Can you think of a person with whom you have unclear or awkward boundaries? How could you clarify those boundaries to yourself and to the other person?

How can you tell that your boundaries are respected?

What threatens good or clear boundaries in your relationships?

Understanding Your Emotional Boundaries

Can you think of a person with whom you are entangled or enmeshed?

Can you maintain a comfortable balance of closeness and distance from others?

Have the boundaries in your relationships been affected by your traumatic experience? If so, how?

Power, Control, and Other People

Do you ever try to control or influence other people? In what situations?

How do you try to control or influence others? What do you do?

As time has passed since your traumatic experience, are you feeling more or less control over people and things around you?

When you feel frightened or threatened around others, do you try to gain some sense of control? How?

Do you use money as a source of power? In what ways?

Do you feel you can openly ask others for what you want? Or do you feel you must try indirectly to control others to get what you want? How do you try to control people indirectly?

Do conflicts and disagreements with other people ever become power struggles? With whom? In what types of relationships?

How do you resolve conflicts?

Symbols of Your Personal Power: Coping with Feelings of Helplessness

When feelings of helplessness arise, you can remind yourself of your strengths and resources through symbols. A symbol for a person who takes Tae Kwan Do might be a black belt, for a teacher it might be his state certificate. Think about what signs, words, licenses (professional or personal), items, or other things might be symbols of your own available knowledge, skills, strengths, and resources. When you are feeling helpless, as everyone does sometimes, think of your symbols of personal power to help ground you and reconnect you with your strengths.

Self-Care Tip

Start by making a list of qualities you like about yourself or that you believe others like about you. Then close your eyes and imagine yourself showing all these good qualities and feeling happy. Where are you as you imagine this? At a party? At work? At home? Outside in nature? Look around the scene in your imagination. What object or image gives you pleasure? Remember that image and bring it to mind whenever you need a boost.

What aspects of your self, your life, or your activities bring you a feeling of strength and empowerment?

What symbols remind you of these aspects of your strengths?

What are the symbols of your strengths in your job?

What are the symbols of your interpersonal strengths?

Is there an object from the world that you can borrow for your own private symbol of strength? It could be a star, a stone, a tree, an image of mother and child. What is it?

Whatever reminds you of your strengths can help you when you feel helpless. You can literally carry this symbol or image around in your pocket, or display it where you can see it often.

SORTING OUT FACTS ABOUT POWER AND CONTROL FROM YOUR REACTIONS: SHADES OF GRAY

Power is not all or nothing. It has degrees and limitations. As we discussed earlier, its meaning can vary along at least two dimensions: ability and effectiveness. Power requires a basic ability to act, but actions may or may not have an effect. Power is action that has an effect. Creating the effect *you* want requires knowledge of yourself. Without self-knowledge, you can expend a great deal of energy to very little effect.

You are the source of your own power; you can learn how to use it. How well do you know yourself? Are you in touch with your thoughts and feelings? Do you respect what you think and feel? Do you know what your abilities are? Do you know how best to use them? You can rate your own current sense of power and control now by circling the appropriate answers in Exercise 6.1.

There are three sections in Exercise 6.1. The abilities in each section of this exercise build on each other. Your source of power is knowledge of yourself. Without this, you will find it difficult to focus your energies effectively. Your abilities for either self-control or having an impact on others will be limited. However, self-knowledge by itself is not enough. To have power, you need to act on the basis of that self-knowledge. To be most effective, you need to know *how* to act and interact with others. Look at your answers. What can you do well? What can you do less well or not at all? Does the problem appear to lie with self-knowledge? With taking action? Or with knowing how to interact with other people?

DO YOU HAVE ENOUGH CONTROL IN YOUR LIFE?

Have will power and force been the only meanings of power and control in your life? We hope you are beginning to see there are other meanings for personal power. How did you rate your degrees of power and influence? The more you circled the lower numbers in Exercise 6.1, the more power and control you experience in your life. Do you have more control than you thought you did? Less? Do you have as much power as you would hope for? The minimum level of power and control that every one needs is

- to control your own actions, to express your own thoughts and feelings
- to have some influence on other people and on your environment—to be able to have an effect or impact

Do you have the ability to control your own actions? To have some influence on others? You have a basic right to express yourself. Do you believe you have this right? Trauma can disrupt or destroy your basic sense of entitle-

EXERCISE 6.1   Rating Your Degree of Power and Influence

Circle the number for how able you think yourself and others are in each of the following situations. When answering, think of recent situations from your day-to-day life. *Do not use a traumatic situation for this or any exercise.*

Circle

1. Extremely able, can almost all the time
2. Very able, can most of the time
3. Moderately able, can often

4. Somewhat able, occasionally can
5. Slightly able, rarely can
6. Not able, have not yet been able

Sources of power/ability—knowing yourself

How able are you	Extremely able					Not able
to know when you feel calm and relaxed	1	2	3	4	5	6
to know when you feel satisfied	1	2	3	4	5	6
to know when you feel dissatisfied	1	2	3	4	5	6
to know when you feel angry	1	2	3	4	5	6
to know when you feel frightened	1	2	3	4	5	6
to know how to comfort yourself when upset	1	2	3	4	5	6
to know when you need help	1	2	3	4	5	6
to know you have a right to your own thoughts and feelings	1	2	3	4	5	6
to know you have a right to express your thoughts and feelings	1	2	3	4	5	6
to know what is most important to you	1	2	3	4	5	6
to know what is less important to you	1	2	3	4	5	6

(continued)

EXERCISE 6.1 (continued)

Power/ability to act—self-control

How able are you	Extremely able				Not able	
to think about your options before you act	1	2	3	4	5	6
to feel angry without acting on it right away	1	2	3	4	5	6
to feel frightened without acting on it right away	1	2	3	4	5	6
to speak when you feel good or satisfied	1	2	3	4	5	6
to clearly say "yes" when you do want something	1	2	3	4	5	6
to speak up when you feel unhappy or dissatisfied	1	2	3	4	5	6
to clearly say "no" when you don't want something	1	2	3	4	5	6
to trust what you really feel and think when another disagrees	1	2	3	4	5	6

Power/ability to act—have an effect on others

How able are you

to know you cannot completely control other people	1	2	3	4	5	6
to respect others' rights to their own thoughts and feelings	1	2	3	4	5	6
to think about your choices before you act to influence others	1	2	3	4	5	6
to ask directly in a positive way for what you want	1	2	3	4	5	6
to listen to others, and check with them that you understand them correctly	1	2	3	4	5	6
to be firm about things most important to you	1	2	3	4	5	6
to be flexible about things less important to you	1	2	3	4	5	6
to be able to see where you have choices	1	2	3	4	5	6

ment to be yourself. During trauma, the consequences of exercising such basic powers can be so terrible that you have no choices, no real ability to act at all. Once out of the traumatic situation, the consequences for exercising your power will be different. The effects of your actions are likely to be different as well, once you are in safer, more respectful relationships.

TRACKING REACTIONS TO BELIEFS ABOUT POWER AND CONTROL

Identifying Your Beliefs about Power and Control

Are you uncomfortable with the current level of control you experience in life? If so, your answers to Exercise 6.1 may help tell you what areas would be helpful for you to work on. Are any of the following areas problems for you?

Do You Know Yourself as Well as You Wish?   Practicing the self-care and self-comfort activities suggested in this workbook are ways to begin connecting with yourself and your inner sources of power and ability. If you have been caring for yourself, you are already on the way to empowering yourself. If you feel your degree of self-knowledge is still low, keep paying attention to your feelings and practicing self-care, and give yourself time to get to know yourself as you now are. Revisit the safety and trust chapters and be sure also to read the first part of Chapter 7 on value and self-esteem.

Do You Have Trouble Expressing Yourself or Believe Self-Expression Won't Make a Difference?   Perhaps you know yourself but believe you have less of a right to express your thoughts and feelings than do others. You may feel that other people are somehow more worthwhile or deserving than you are and that you should take a back seat. How did you answer the last four statements in the first section of Exercise 6.1? Did you disagree that you have the right to your own thoughts, feelings, and their expression? Are you able to say no or to hold to what you feel and think when another disagrees? Do you have trouble saying "no" when you really want to say "no"? If this could be a problem for you, be sure to also read Chapter 7 on valuing yourself. That chapter goes into deeper detail on the issues and possibilities surrounding this problem.

Do You Feel You Don't Have Any Impact on Others?   This question does not ask if you feel totally able to control others or always get your own way. The answer to that question is that you can't. You can't control others and you can't always get your own way. This is the reality of life. However, you have power to do other things, if you can learn where to focus your efforts. Start by focusing within yourself, on what you think, feel, and want, with how you act and interact with others. By doing this you can increase your abilities, skills, and your sense of power.

Learning skills and abilities is important but it may not be enough. Your beliefs about power and control may get in your way. Think now of a particular time you experienced a problem with power or control issues. Perhaps a particular situation came to mind as you read about one of three areas of power and control, or when you completed Exercise 6.1. Use that specific situation in Exercise 6.2 to see if you can identify an underlying belief you have about power and control.

Let's look at how Maureen completed this exercise. She had survived sexual abuse. She now had a job and an apartment, but she had difficulty feeling a sense of personal power in her life and in her relationships. She often felt especially helpless after talking with her mother. Just the other day, she confided in her mother that she'd been thinking of taking a course at the community college to see if she could handle college-level work. Her mother responded by saying, "Why would you want to do that? Your sister is getting along fine without any college. Wouldn't it mean a lot of extra work? I can't imagine anybody in their right mind wanting to go back to school if they didn't have to." Maureen has felt bad since the conversation. She feels it's hopeless to think about taking the course. When she came to Exercise 6.2, she wrote the following for the situation:

How can I take this college course when my mother doesn't think I should?

Maureen looked at the first question, which asked what this situation said about her. She wrote down what immediately popped into her head:

I am a little weakling.

Maureen then had to consider what that statement said about her. She wrote

I should be strong enough to do what I want regardless of what Mom thinks.

EXERCISE 6.2   Identifying Beliefs about Power and Control

In this exercise, we ask you to describe a recent situation in which you had a problem with power and control. *Do not use a traumatic situation for this exercise.* If you cannot think of a recent situation, look at your answers to Exercise 6.1. Did you rate any items as a 4, 5, or 6? Are these areas in which you wish you were more able? Use a (nontrau-matic) problem situation that comes to mind when you think of those items. In the first line below, describe the situation. Next, write what you think that situation says about you. After you write a response, look at what you wrote. Then write what that says about you. Continue answering the questions by looking at your immediately preced-ing answer. Then for each following question, think mainly about what you wrote as an answer for the question immediately above it.

Situation:

_____

_____

What does this say or mean about me?

_____

_____

Looking at what I just wrote, what does that say or mean about me?

_____

_____

What does that, in turn, say or mean about me?

_____

_____

Looking at all the above, can I drawn any conclusions about me?

_____

_____

Adapted with permission from Dennis Greenberger and Christine Padesky, *Mind Over Mood: Change How You Feel by Changing the Way You Think.* New York: Guilford Press, 1995

What did that say about Maureen?

> But I'm not. I can't bear to make my mother unhappy. She'll be disappointed in me. Then I will feel even more terrible; I'll be a bad daughter.

Looking at all the above, can Maureen draw any conclusions about herself and power/control? She wrote

> I can't win. No matter what I do, I'll feel bad. There are no good choices.

Given what Maureen has written, it makes sense that she feels powerless and out of control. But thinking about this was just like hitting her head against the same old brick wall. Doing this exercise made her feel even more hopeless, at first. But if Maureen can bring herself to look more carefully at the brick wall, she might discover a way through it, or at least a way around it. She might even discover that the brick wall protects her in some ways that she might not want to give up.

Evaluating How a Belief Helps and Hinders You

In Exercise 6.3, we ask you to think about the advantages and disadvantages of the belief you identified on the last line of Exercise 6.2. For Maureen, the belief was "I can't win. There are no good choices." She could see there were lots of disadvantages to believing she was caught in a no-win situation. But what could she do about it? She couldn't quite believe there would be any advantages, but she decided to go along and fill out the exercise anyway.

Any belief will have both benefits and drawbacks. You need to weigh the pros and cons of each of your beliefs. Exercise 6.3 helps you do that. If you wish, you can also choose another belief that you have identified. Maureen expressed a number of other beliefs in her Exercise 6.2. For example, she believes she is a "weakling" and not "strong enough." Maureen decided to look further at the belief "I can't win. There are no good choices."

When you finish answering the questions, take a look at the exercise as a whole. Are your answers more toward helping you or hindering you? If the belief hinders more than helps, you might want to question how accurate it really is.

When Maureen finished this exercise, she was surprised to find that the beliefs did have some positive effects. It certainly simplified her life and

EXERCISE 6.3   How Does This Belief Help and Hinder Me?

Most beliefs have both advantages and disadvantages. Consider those for the belief you identified in the last line of Exercise 6.2. Write down the belief in the space below, then circle how helpful or hindering the belief is for each question.

Belief: _____

Circle

1. Extremely helpful	4. Not at all helpful
2. Very helpful	5. Gets in my way
3. Moderately helpful	6. Gets in my way a lot

	Extremely helpful			**Gets in my way a lot**		
1. How helpful is this belief?	1	2	3	4	5	6
2. How calming is this belief?	1	2	3	4	5	6
3. How flexible is this belief?	1	2	3	4	5	6
4. How safe does this belief make me feel?	1	2	3	4	5	6
5. Does this belief help me understand myself?	1	2	3	4	5	6
6. Does this belief give me hope?	1	2	3	4	5	6
7. How essential is the belief to my survival?	1	2	3	4	5	6
8. How well does this belief help me cope?	1	2	3	4	5	6
9. Does the belief help me make sense of the world?	1	2	3	4	5	6
10. Does this belief help me make decisions?	1	2	3	4	5	6
11. Does this belief help me know what I need for myself?	1	2	3	4	5	6

made decision-making easy—at least about this course. But it also made her very hopeless. It did not help her know what she needed for herself.

Pinpointing Problem Areas to Think Through Further

As a next step, think about your answers in Exercises 6.2. As you look at them, consider the following two questions:

1. Do the degree and range of your powers and abilities circled in Exercise 6.1 match your sense of power by the conclusion of Exercise 6.2?

2. Can you see all-or-nothing thinking at work in any of your responses in Exercise 6.2?

Maureen felt very powerless by the end of Exercise 6.2. But when she looked at how she'd filled out Exercise 6.1 she found she had circled quite a number of items as at least "somewhat able." Her own ratings in Exercise 6.1 showed that she probably wasn't as powerless as she felt in the situation with her mother. She certainly *felt* powerless; perhaps the way she felt wasn't completely accurate.

When she looked for any all-or-nothing thinking in how she'd described the situation with her mother, at first she didn't see any. The statements all felt so true to her: "I can't win." "No matter what I do, I'll feel bad," and "There are no good choices." As she thought about it further, however, she realized that she only saw two choices and those were either/or choices. She couldn't win *because* that meant her mother had to lose. This is how all-or-nothing thinking often looks. If you only see two choices, and they are opposites or either/or choices, then all-or-nothing thinking is probably at work.

If Maureen took the course, as she wanted, she believed her mother would be hurt and disappointed and that meant Maureen would be a bad daughter. But doing what her mother wanted meant denying her own needs and wants. Winning versus losing is just another version of all-or-nothing thinking. When it comes to power and control issues, all-or-nothing thinking often takes the form of win versus lose, us versus them, me versus you. But these are not the only available choices. Maureen also seems to be confused about the boundaries between herself and her mother. Her mother may also be confused.

As you look at your own answers to the exercises so far, remind yourself about the sources and limitations of power. You might feel powerless because you are trying to control entirely something that you can't. You may also feel powerless because you can't control something that you can learn at least partly to control. For example, in the last chapter we talked about Bonnie who did not trust herself to talk about her feelings without crying. She felt powerless to shut down the wave of emotion that would sweep through her and make her cry. When Bonnie got to this chapter, she was surprised to read that what we truly think and feel inside cannot be completely controlled. She believed she was weak because she could not stop the wave of emotion and her tears, but she was simply human. She could, in fact, gain more control over her crying if she learned to listen to the emotion rather than try to shut it down completely.

Time Out for Self-Care

If completing the exercises so far has overwhelmed or upset you in any way, take time out for yourself. Talk to others or try the relaxation exercises or other self-care activities suggested elsewhere in this book.

Taking Stock

Do you feel comfortable with the level of control you have in your own life? Pause now to consider what you need and want. Do you want to continue working on issues of power and control? Do you want to put this work aside for now? Feel free to stop now if you choose. If you prefer to work on other issues right now, feel free to do so. Exercise 6.4 (see page 212) asks you to take stock of where you are in your work on power and control. Fill this out as a record, then move on to do whatever you need to do right now. If you check item 5, then continue on in this chapter by reading the next section.

EXERCISE 6.4 Taking Stock of Your Work on Power and Control

Consider what you think and feel right now. Do you wish to take a break from this work? Do you wish to continue? Please check the statement that describes your situation right now.

_____ 1. My beliefs about power and control are fine. I do not need to think them through further. I am comfortable with the level of control I feel over my own actions.

_____ 2. My beliefs about power, control, and other people are fine. I do not need to think them through further. I am comfortable with the level of power and influence I have with other people in my life.

_____ 3. There are situations in which I might not feel a comfortable level of personal power and self-control, but I do not want to think through my beliefs about power and control right now. I can come back to this work whenever I wish.

_____ 4. There are situations and ways in which I might not feel a comfortable level of personal power and influence with others, but I do not want to think through my beliefs about power and control right now. I can come back to this work whenever I wish.

_____ 5. I am beginning to think about why some of my beliefs about control and power do not work. I can continue to work on these beliefs, but I want to move slowly and carefully. I can stop this work at any time.

_____ 6. I am ready to think through a belief about power and control.

If you checked 5 or 6 above, write down here any beliefs that you may wish to work further on now or at some future time:

_____

_____

_____

_____

_____

_____

_____

THINKING THROUGH A BELIEF ABOUT POWER AND CONTROL

The exercises in the rest of this chapter help you look more closely at problems you may have with power and control. The exercises ask you to think about times since the trauma when you have felt helpless, out of control, and without choices. *Do not use a traumatic experience in any of these exercises.* Remember to take care of yourself as you answer the questions. Be sure to pay attention to your feelings. Stop if trauma memories or emotions are triggered or if you might be emotionally overwhelmed. Take time out for self-care whenever you need it; caring for yourself is an exercise in personal power.

Choosing Beliefs to Work On

Make a list below of the beliefs you have identified so far that you would like to think through more completely. Perhaps you have none, one, or several. Write down any that you have below:

_____

_____

_____

For *each* belief you have written above, complete the questions in Exercise 6.5 (see pages 214–215). This exercise asks you to review some of the same ground you covered in earlier exercises, but takes you a step further. Start with a situation in which the belief about power and control influenced your experience. You can use the same situation you used for identifying that belief or choose another situation in which you felt helpless or out of control.

Sort Out the Facts of What Happened

Maureen decided to think more about her difficulty with her mother so she used the same situation as she had in Exercise 6.2. For the facts of the situation, Maureen wrote

> I told my mother I was thinking about taking a course. She said that nobody in their right mind would want to go back to school if they didn't have to. So, I just shut up and didn't say anything else.

EXERCISE 6.5   Steps for Thinking Through a Belief about Power and Control

The belief you wish to think through:

_____

Sort Out the Facts of What Happened

Think of a particular situation in which this belief may have been a problem. You can use the same situation you used to identify the belief, or use another situation in which power or control was an issue. Describe the facts. What happened? What was the sequence of events?

Sort Out the Meaning the Facts Have for You

How did you interpret this situation? What did it mean to you?

Identify the Underlying Belief

What lesson did you draw from it about yourself? About other people?

When did you start believing this about yourself or others? Was this incident the first time? If not, when and how do you remember first learning this lesson?

Evaluate the Pros and Cons of the Belief

How does believing this make you feel about yourself or others? What does it make you think about yourself or others?

How does believing this help you or protect you?

How does believing this hold you back or get in your way?

Imagine Alternative Meanings for the Same Facts

Look back at your description of what happened (the first question above). Are there other ways to interpret what happened? What else could the situation mean? Is there an alternative meaning that would fit the facts of what happened? If so, what is it?

Evaluate the Pros and Cons of the Alternative Meaning

What positive feelings do you have when you think about this alternative meaning?

What negative feelings do you have when you think about this alternative meaning?

Consider How to Check the Accuracy of These Beliefs

How could you test to see whether or not your belief is true?

How high is the risk if you test the truth of what you believe? How dangerous would it be?

What good things might happen if you test the truth of what you believe?

Put the Process in Perspective

Will testing the belief matter 10 years from now? Would it help or hinder you in the future?

Sort Out the Meaning the Facts Have for You

Maureen was then asked to write down what this situation meant to her. She wrote

I must be weird to want to go back to school. If I do it, my mother will be unhappy and I'll be a bad daughter.

Identify the Underlying Belief

Maureen then was asked to take the meaning one step further to state the lesson she saw in this experience. She wrote

When my mother and I think differently, I can't win. There are no good choices.

The next question asked Maureen to identify when she had first learned this lesson. She realized that she'd learned it as a child. A good daughter did what her mother wanted. When her mother was unhappy with her it meant she was bad. When she did something her mother didn't approve of, she felt terrible. As she thought about this, she realized that this wasn't a big problem when she was a child; in those days, she could "win" by being a good daughter and doing what her mother wanted. It was only since she grew up and starting having her own ideas that the situation became "no win" for her.

Evaluate the Pros and Cons of the Belief

The next three questions in the exercise asked Maureen how the belief made her feel about herself, how it helped her, and also how it held her back. The belief made Maureen feel powerless, but it was generally easy and calming to give in to what her mother wanted all the time. It was upsetting not to give in. While it helped her understand herself as a good daughter, it also made her feel hopeless much of the time. The belief did not help her know what she needed for herself. In fact, the belief worked against her knowing that or acting on it. Thinking about how the belief generally held her back rather than helped her gave Maureen an incentive to think about other ways to interpret what had happened between her and her mother.

Imagine an Alternative Interpretation for the Same Facts

The exercise next asked Maureen to look again at the facts of the situation and try to imagine an alternative interpretation. She found it helpful at this point to go over some of the earlier parts of this chapter. Exercise 6.1 and the section on "The Sources and Limitations of Personal Power and Control" in particular were helpful in reminding her of what she could control and what she could not. Maureen had exercised power when she'd expressed her thoughts to her mother about taking the course. But when her mother wasn't very positive, Maureen began to feel as if she really did not have any power at all. She saw that part of the trouble was described in one of the items in Exercise 6.1: "to trust what you really feel and think when another disagrees." The items in the third section of the exercise gave her even more to think about. She knew very well that she could not completely control other people. She felt she had little control over other people, such as her mother. What she had trouble believing was that others, especially her mother, could not control her. Wasn't it a mother's role to control her children? On the other hand, Maureen wasn't a child anymore. In theory, she knew that people had a right to feel and think differently from each other. In practice, when it came to someone close such as her mother, she was afraid she would permanently damage the relationship. Another part of Maureen's dilemma was feeling she could not be "good" and also have enough control in her life. Maureen will find more to think about on this issue when she reads the next chapter on self-esteem.

It was hard for Maureen to think of an alternative meaning to the incident with her mother but she finally came up with one. Perhaps it was really about how much her mother had disliked being in school. Why should her mother care that much if she herself didn't have to go back to school?

Evaluate the Pros and Cons of the Alternative Meaning

When Maureen thought a bit about this alternative meaning, she felt some hope return. If her mother wasn't a problem, then she would be free to take the course. On the other hand, what if her belief was right and her mother was angry or unhappy with her? That would be painful. She'd be back where she started.

Consider How to Check the Accuracy of the Belief

At first, the only way Maureen could think of to test the accuracy of her belief was to take the course. But this felt very high risk. Fortunately, there are almost always smaller, lower risk steps to check out a belief. The simplest but not always the most obvious of these ways is for Maureen to ask her mother what she meant. Was she telling Maureen not to take the course? The worst thing that could happen would be for her mother to agree that this is what she meant. If this happened, Maureen didn't have to do anything else. She could just say, "That's what I thought you probably meant, but I wasn't sure." Almost any other response from her mother would be a good thing.

Maureen decided to go ahead and ask her mother directly. She thought ahead about what she was going to ask, and then she called her mother. She said

> Remember last time we talked and I mentioned that course I was thinking of taking? I thought you were saying that I shouldn't go back to school. Is that what you meant?

Maureen did this and her mother's answer surprised her. Her mother said,

> I didn't mean you *shouldn't* take the course. You should do what you want. But it's just not something I'd want to do. I'm afraid you are going to find out too late you don't really want to do it either.

Maureen still believed that her mother preferred her not to take the course, but there was more flexibility than she had anticipated. Her mother seemed to be backing off a bit in her disapproval. Maureen was still afraid there might be a high emotional price to pay for taking the course if her mother really didn't want her to. After a few days, she decided to ask her mother another question. Her question to her mother was

> How would you feel about me if I went ahead and took the course?

When Maureen asked this, it was her mother's turn to be surprised.

> I didn't realize how important this seems to be to you. If you took the course, I'd be worried that you wouldn't enjoy it, but it's your decision. All I meant was that I wouldn't want to do it.

The message that Maureen heard this time was that the course was much more important to Maureen than to her mother. Maureen was right to pick up that her mother didn't understand or like the idea of Maureen taking the course, but now it seemed that the whole thing wasn't all that important to her mother. It surprised Maureen that her mother had not known how big a deal it really was to her.

Put the Process in Perspective

It can be difficult to see something from another perspective when immersed in your own experience and feelings. Taking the time to think carefully through other possible explanations and perspectives can turn up surprising information. Although it can be difficult to know how, exactly, to go about collecting more information, the following steps may help. Gathering additional information, paying closer attention, and asking questions, at times can uncover pleasantly unexpected information and possibilities.

WEIGHING THE EVIDENCE ON BELIEFS ABOUT POWER AND CONTROL

For Maureen the process of thinking through her belief and then checking it out moved along very fast for this situation. She didn't need exercises on brainstorming ideas or the list of baby steps to help her move through the process. That may also be your experience for some situations and if it works for you, that's fine. For other situations, you may need the exercises to help you come up with low-risk ways to collect evidence, help you rank those ideas by risk, and help you keep track of the evidence you collect.

Brainstorm Ideas for Collecting Evidence

If you have identified a belief about power and control that you might consider testing, brainstorm for ideas on how to collect evidence on its accuracy. Use Exercise 6.6 (see page 220) if you need to. Consider the following kinds of low-risk ways to collect evidence:

1. Notice or observe events, actions, or people.
2. Watch others' reactions to an event, action, or person.
3. Notice when you are already carrying out actions that produce evidence about your belief.
4. Ask friends questions about their reactions to a third person or event.
5. When it feels safe enough, take a small action with a safe friend that tests the belief and see how the friend reacts.

**EXERCISE 6.6   Brainstorm Ideas for Collecting Evidence
on a Belief**

Create a list of rough ideas for collecting evidence on a belief. The goal is to come up
with some low-risk ways to collect evidence, but be prepared that the first ideas you
have may be high risk. Write them down to get them out of the way. You do not need
to carry out *any* of the ideas you write down. You will screen these ideas later and discard any you choose. Begin by writing down a belief and an alternative interpretation
on which you want to collect evidence. In the blank space below write down any and
all ideas that come to mind for how to do this.

Belief: _____

Alternative interpretation: _____

Rank Ideas by Lowest Risk First

When you have brainstormed a number of specific ways you could collect evidence, the next step is to rank them according to risk. You can do this using the blank form in Exercise 6.7 (see page 222). In the spaces at the top of the form, write down your existing belief, and an alternative interpretation. Then, on your rough brainstorming list, review all the ideas you have written down and find the one with the lowest risk. Remember, you do *not* have to carry out *any* of the ideas you've written down. But if you did decide to try one, what would be the consequences? For which ideas are the worst consequences not that bad? Which idea seems the easiest and the safest to carry out? If you don't have any easy and safe ideas, you need to go back and do more brainstorming. Otherwise, write down the lowest risk idea at the top of the baby steps list directly under "Least Feared Actions/Observations." Then cross that idea off your rough list. Out of the remaining ideas on your rough brainstorming list, find the one that is now lowest risk. Write that on the second line of the baby steps list and cross it off your rough brainstorming list. Continue selecting the lowest risk idea from among those you have not yet crossed off the brainstorming list. At some point, you may find that the only ideas left have bad consequences. These ideas are not baby steps. High-risk ways to collect evidence do not belong on the baby steps list. You don't have to fill the list. If you have enough low-risk ideas to fill all 10 lines for baby steps, rank only the low- to reasonable-risk ideas you can safely imagine yourself doing.

Carry Out Lowest Risk Ways to Collect Evidence

When you are ready, you can begin to carry out the observations and tests you have listed as baby steps.

Record and Weigh the Evidence for and against the Belief

We enclose two sheets for recording evidence. Exercise 6.8 (page 223) and Exercise 6.9 (page 224) are basically the same except that one is for recording evidence of your existing belief and the other for evidence on the alternative meaning. Remember, you can stop this work at any time and come back to it at any time.

EXERCISE 6.7   Baby Steps for Testing a Belief about Power and Control

In the first blanks below, write down the belief you are thinking of testing and an alternative interpretation. When you have brainstormed ideas for possible ways to collect evidence on a belief, rank those ideas by risk, starting with the lowest risk ways. List only ways that are within a reasonable risk. *Do not list any high-risk ways to collect evidence.*

Belief: _____

Alternative interpretation: _____

Least Feared Actions/Observations

_____

_____

_____

_____

_____

_____

_____

_____

_____

Most Feared Actions/Observations

EXERCISE 6.8   What Evidence Do I Have about the Existing Belief?

What evidence do you already have about the accuracy of your existing belief? What facts, words, or actions support the belief? What facts, words, or actions indicate the belief is inaccurate? Write those down below.

Belief: _____

What facts or evidence support this belief as accurate?

1. _____

2. _____

3. _____

What facts or evidence indicate this belief is not accurate?

1. _____

2. _____

3. _____

How sure are you that this belief is accurate? Mark how sure on the following scale. Use the second evaluation scale later to check on changes in your beliefs in light of new evidence.

Date: _____

Accurate   Inaccurate

_____

100%   50%   0%

Date: _____

Accurate   Inaccurate

_____

100%   50%   0%

EXERCISE 6.9   What Evidence Do I Have
about the Alternative Meaning?

What evidence do you already have about the accuracy of the alternative meaning? What facts, words, or actions support the alternative meaning? What facts, words, or actions indicate the alternative meaning is inaccurate? Write those down below.

Alternative meaning: _____

What facts or evidence support this interpretation as accurate?

1. _____
2. _____
3. _____

What facts or evidence indicate this interpretation is not accurate?

1. _____
2. _____
3. _____

How sure are you that this interpretation is accurate? Mark how sure on the following scale. Use the second evaluation scale later to check on changes in your beliefs in light of new evidence.

Date: _____

Accurate   Inaccurate

_____

100%   50%   0%

Date: _____

Accurate   Inaccurate

_____

100%   50%   0%

Many of the lowest risk ways to collect evidence on a belief involve observation. Carrying this out can be trickier than you think. We tend to notice the facts that support our beliefs and miss those that do not. For this reason, you need to test an existing belief and an alternative interpretation together, at the same time. Do the facts you notice apply to both beliefs or only one and not the other? In collecting observations as evidence, you need to pay attention to the facts of what actually happens. This means being able to sort out the facts from your interpretations, thoughts, and feelings about it.

SUMMARIZING YOUR WORK ON POWER AND CONTROL

Consider now what you need for yourself. You can put this workbook aside for now, or you can continue to work on it as you choose. You may move on to the next chapter in the workbook or you can revisit parts of this or earlier chapters. Feel free to identify other beliefs about power and control, evaluate them, and test how accurate they may be. When you are ready to stop your work on power and control for the time being, complete Exercise 6.10 (see page 226) as a summary of your work. You can return to issues of power and control at any time. Review this summary when you come back. It will give you a sense of where you are and what else you might want to work on.

Despite how strongly you may feel, you are not helpless. You are not powerless. A sense of personal power is there for you to find when you are ready. It does not have to be violent or coercive. It can be creative and constructive. This choice is in your power. The basis of your personal power lies in how well you know yourself, your feelings and abilities as well as your limitations.

Do you remember how it feels to be capable? Do you remember a sense of power in the first time you rode a bike? Power lies in your abilities.

There is power in knowing what you feel and think.

There is power in knowing how to comfort yourself.

There is power is expressing yourself.

There is power in the skills with which you express yourself.

There is power in your knowledge of your limitations.

EXERCISE 6.10   Summarizing Your Work on Power and Control

I have identified the following beliefs about power and control:

I can think of the following alternative meanings:

I have carried out the following steps (mark with X); or I would like in the future to carry out the following steps (mark with *):

_____ Make a list of what evidence might confirm and/or contradict the existing belief.

_____ Organize the list of evidence from least feared/least risky to collect to most feared/most risky to collect.

_____ Carry out the least feared/least risky way to collect evidence.

_____ Keep a record of the evidence collected—both pro and con.

List here any evidence collected—what did you see or do, and how did it turn out? Continue adding to this list over time, as you become aware of additional evidence.

$\mathcal{V}$ALUING YOURSELF AND OTHERS

YOUR NEED FOR ESTEEM: The need to value what you feel, think, and believe; the need to value others.

EVERY NEW ADJUSTMENT is a crisis in self-esteem.

—Eric Hoffer, *The Ordeal of Change*

HOW TRAUMA CAN AFFECT SELF-ESTEEM

You need to value yourself and others. When you do both, you are more likely to have a sense of belonging, connection, and control. Trauma, whether a single or repeated event, can devastate how positively you feel about yourself and other people. When you have self-esteem, you have faith in yourself, think about yourself in positive ways and generally feel understood. You expect others to treat you with respect and take you seriously. When you lack self-esteem, you can feel bad, damaged, worthless, or evil. You may also feel that other people are this way.

Following a trauma, you may feel on top of the world one day and at the very bottom the next. You may feel a rush of warm, positive feelings for another person, or people in general, but then become convinced that people are fundamentally bad. You may feel so disappointed in yourself after trauma, that you no longer feel a basic sense of value or worth. These enormous fluctuations in your mood and how you feel can leave you feeling as though there is no solid foundation supporting you and no comforting sense that you know how you will feel or see things from moment to moment.

Traumatic events are particularly damaging to self-esteem if you were treated as worthless by others. You may have absorbed the negative messages of the perpetrators, and now see yourself as unworthy of love, attention, praise, or reward. If your family and friends can't support, accept, or understand you, your self-esteem may also suffer. You may begin to wonder if you are worthy of being cared for in these ways. Children are particularly vulnerable to these messages. They have limited experience and generally believe what their parents and other important adults tell them.

❧ *Nettie's father constantly told her that she was worthless. As a child, she depended on her father who was stronger and more experienced. His messages about her faults and shortcomings undermined her sense of self-esteem. As an adult, she continues to struggle with the effect of believing these negative messages that she heard growing up. Remembering the specific things she most likes about herself helps.*

When we hear negative messages about ourselves, we usually feel shame. Feelings of shame often come with thoughts of our failings. As we discussed in Chapter 1, it is not uncommon for trauma survivors to have strong and upsetting emotional reactions. Shame is among the most devastating of these emotions because it can have such a powerful negative impact on self-esteem. It can also make it more difficult to share feelings and experiences with others.

Shame and Self-Esteem

Everyone feels shame from time to time because we are all human and imperfect. Healthy shame is the emotional recognition of these human failings and imperfections. Healthy shame does not wipe out a sense of self-worth but coexists with it and can motivate us to try harder. However, shame can become exaggerated, unbearable, and paralyzing. Such exaggerated feelings of shame can undermine or completely block recognition of your own value. You may wish to hide, disappear, or apologize for who you are.

Remember that emotions such as shame or fear are not necessarily accurate for the current circumstances. You can feel afraid without being in any immediate danger. You can also feel worthless even when you have great value and many strengths. This chapter is designed to help remind you of what is good and valuable about yourself. So take your time. Go slow and put this work aside whenever you feel you need to. You may want to revisit Chapter 2, particularly its section on coping with negative feelings. Taking care of yourself is a crucial step in rebuilding self-esteem.

Responsibility, Anger, and Blame

One reason trauma survivors may feel overwhelmed with shame is that they feel responsible in some way for what happened to them. It is not uncommon for survivors of various kinds of trauma to think, "Why didn't I fight harder, run faster, yell louder, hold on tighter?" You may feel that you failed because you couldn't protect yourself or others from what happened. These questions can quickly turn into self-criticisms, setting in motion a vicious cycle. It can feel like a runaway roller coaster, difficult to slow down or stop. As you make ordinary mistakes, you criticize yourself more and more harshly. You may believe that if only you didn't make mistakes, you would feel good about yourself. It is human to err; no one is perfect and total control is impossible. Self-criticism and impossible standards only erode self-esteem further. Accepting your foibles and imperfections is, in fact, an integral step toward self-acceptance and self-esteem. It may surprise you that sharing your frailties creates your strongest bonds with others. It is possible to feel good about yourself without being perfect, just as it is possible to have control without being in total control. In fact, forgiving yourself for your trauma goes hand-in-hand with accepting that you were not in control of what happened.

During the traumatic event, the terror of the moment probably shocked you into confusion, paralysis, or a total focus on survival and the effort to anticipate what was going to happen next. You did what was possible for you to do in the moment. You may have come face to face with your own limitations. It is extremely painful to accept a loss of control in your life. At times, people cling to the belief that they can control things when, in fact, they cannot. Harsh self-blame can feel safer and less devastating than accepting that there are things not under your control. If you believe you could control something which you truly could not, it can damage the way you feel about yourself. You may lose sight of what you still can control.

Feeling very angry at yourself is another way you might blame yourself for a traumatic experience. Feeling angry at ourselves or others can sometimes keep us from more uncomfortable feelings such as shame, sadness, or hurt.

> ❖ *It took years after his abuse before Mark could begin to realize how angry he sometimes got at other people. He had learned that anger was explosive and dangerous. For a long time, it seemed too risky to feel angry at others. Instead it actually felt safer to feel intense anger toward himself. During these times, he felt his anger was in charge. It took him a while to realize he also felt ashamed at these times—and that he also felt tremendous emotional pain like he felt when abused as a child.*

Keeping the focus of anger, blame, and shame on yourself may also be a way to protect a valued relationship with someone else. Anger or self-blame may seem more manageable than the intense loss and grief that would arise if you fully realized what someone cherished did to you.

> ❖ *Fran had a clear sense of the abuse she had endured from her father. Her memories of her mother were vague. She felt generally uncomfortable about her mother, but she discounted the feelings and instead felt guilty for even questioning the relationship. It took time for her to face the knowledge that her mother had also been abusive. Doubting herself allowed her to believe, at least for a while, that at least one parent had treated her with love and respect.*

Withdrawing from Others

When you don't feel good about yourself, you may cope by withdrawing from others. You may isolate yourself physically and not see much of other people. You can also isolate yourself emotionally. You may allow people to know only certain aspects of who you are. You may have difficulty letting go or being spontaneous. You may remain guarded so that no one can get close to you. If others get close, you may fear they'll learn of your "badness." You may feel, "If they really get to know me, they won't like me," or "They like me but they really don't know me." These thoughts are barriers to trust and intimacy in your relationships.

> ❖ *Sharon, a survivor of sexual abuse from multiple perpetrators, deliberately harms herself on a regular basis. Her last two friendships have been with*

*other women who are also survivors. After they got to know Sharon, they
also began to cut themselves. Sharon believes that she is responsible for their
cutting and has resolved to develop no new friendships. She fears that anyone who becomes her friend could begin to hurt herself as well.*

Withdrawing from others may seem protective, but it prevents any chance
for real closeness.

Valuing Other People

How did you answer questions about trusting others in Chapter 5? If you
find yourself distrustful of others, perhaps you expect them to be dishonest,
selfish, or uncaring. Perhaps you feel they are not deserving of your respect
or value. Issues of trust and esteem for others are connected. Traumatic
events resulting from the action or inaction of another person can bring you
face-to-face with the worst in human nature. Personal experience of this can
lead you to believe that human nature is basically evil. Even when others
treat you kindly, you may doubt their motives.

> ❀ *Nick found himself developing a deepening connection with his therapist.
> This was difficult and frightening because part of him believed that the
> only reason the therapist would want to get closer would be to use it against
> him in some way eventually. These feelings, based on his past experiences
> made him want to run away.*

Trauma can disrupt the good faith you have in another person or, more
generally, in humanity. You may find yourself wondering about other people.
What don't you yet know about them? Could they harm you or someone
else? Trauma can teach you the hard truth about how terrible people can be.
But does this mean that *all* people are *always* terrible?

Sometimes the way you feel about others is linked to the way you feel
about yourself. If you feel you must be perfect to have worth and value, you
will probably hold others to the same standards. If you fear that you are fundamentally bad, unworthy, or undeserving, you may see those aspects in others. Over time in any relationship, however, it is inevitable that people will
let each other down. We are only human. When this happens you may feel
great pain. However, when you feel generally good about yourself, you are

more likely to forgive others, just as you can more easily forgive yourself. It is possible to feel good about others even if they sometimes let you down.

Trauma Survivors Speak about Self-Esteem

• There are several definitions under esteem in the dictionary, but the one that best applies is the first: to regard highly or favorably; regard with respect or admiration. The synonym is appreciate. Self-esteem is defined as self-respect. Self-esteem can also be thought of as self-liking or self loving. . . . Esteem and self-esteem are so intertwined as to be inseparable. If one is lacking, the other is impossible to achieve.

• A good parent sends the message that the child only has to do one thing to be loved: she only has to *be*. Just *be*. Later the rules of living can be learned, how people should treat each other, how behavior can be good or bad, what consequences are and what being responsible means. But all of that flows from the basic feeling of being totally accepted as a person and valued for just existing in the world.

• Esteem is feeling good about yourself, feeling worthwhile. Esteem is feeling comfortable with yourself, accepting even your flaws. It's okay to have flaws. Esteem is not fearing everything. It is trying new things and saying things for yourself rather than what someone else wants to hear. Esteem is self-love.

WHAT CAN VALUE AND ESTEEM MEAN?

It is normal for people to judge others and judge themselves. We usually evaluate our own behaviors by the standard of how we would most like to be. We usually judge others by the standard of how we would most like them to be. When we fall short of our own expectations in everyday life, healthy shame can motivate us to try harder without destroying our basic sense of worth. When our basic sense of self-esteem is damaged or destroyed, we need to consider what fundamental things give value to any person. You may think you know what a "good" or a "bad" person is. But different people would probably mean different things by these words. Most ways of evaluating people are not absolute. Each human being is, in fact, complicated and variable.

You are a complex assortment of strengths and weaknesses. Each of your individual aspects has its own value. Taken as a whole, each human individual is neither good nor bad, worthy nor unworthy, but rather a complicated mix of abilities and inabilities, strengths and weaknesses, talents and inadequacies, ignorance and expertise. What, then, does it mean to be worthy, to have value, to merit esteem—for yourself and for others? The answer is complicated because the meaning of *value* or *worth* can itself shift and change. For example, is a person who takes his time making decisions thorough or indecisive? Is his behavior a strength or a weakness? Both answers could be correct depending on the situation. There is no single right answer. Rather, the answer depends, at least, on the following conditions:

- Who is doing the valuing?
- What is the overall situation?
- What standards are being used?

An ability to work on your own can be a weakness in a situation demanding teamwork, but the same characteristic can be a strength if the situation requires you to work out of your home. Behavior called flexible by one person can be called wishy-washy by someone else. Different people can judge value differently and these judgments can all be valid. This is because value is usually based on what the evaluator wants, and this may or may not be the same thing you want or need. You can be caught between what you need for yourself, and what someone else wants from you. Different people may want different, even contradictory, things from you at the same time. It is difficult to value yourself when no one else does, but if you base your self-worth only on how others judge you, it is based on shifting sands. Only *you* know what you want and need. Only *you* can know what is important for you. This is why you need to have a firm sense of your own values.

❈ *After years in a verbally abusive marriage, Marshall felt as though nothing he did was ever right. He felt bad about himself because he always fell short of his wife's expectations, and even started feeling uncertain about his skills at work. It was difficult for him to believe that anyone valued his contributations when he felt so devalued in his marriage.*

Your self-esteem depends on what *you* think and feel about yourself, how *you* value yourself. In the last chapter we said that empowerment starts with recognizing and respecting what you need and want. Self-esteem, like power, also has its source in knowing your needs and wants.

What Is of Value to You?

To value something or someone is to realize that it is important to you. Importance by itself isn't always enough; unless you are aware of that importance, you may not value it. Being alive is important, but it is also easy to take for granted. Sometimes, it is not until life is threatened that we fully realize how much we value it. To value something is to appreciate how important it is to you.

Value is not always a fixed quality. It can fluctuate, growing or shrinking as situations change. The value of eating fluctuates with how hungry you are. It is never completely unimportant because you need to eat to live. On the other hand, eating too much of the wrong things can begin to endanger your health. In that situation, eating less can become more important for your overall health. Anything that helps meet your basic needs is important to you, whether you realize it or not. Realizing it, however, can make it easier for you to get those needs met. This is especially important when two or more of your needs appear to compete with each other. Recognizing this can allow you to balance them so that you can have enough of each.

A poor sense of your own worth is a barrier to realizing the importance of your basic needs. You may believe that you are fundamentally undeserving. You may believe that other people's needs and wishes have more weight and importance than your own. You may believe the judgments of others have more value than your own. If you feel this way, it might help to understand better the distinction between rights and rewards.

The Difference between Rights and Rewards

One lesson that survivors sometimes draw from trauma is that they do not deserve respect, do not deserve to be happy, or even do not deserve to have their basic needs met. If you feel this way, it can help to ask yourself how deserving is measured. Who decides what is and isn't deserving? Where does your personal sense of worth come from?

If you believe you are not a deserving person, you were probably treated by another in this way. You may have come to believe that life itself, respect, and the fulfillment of basic needs are special rewards that must be earned. Many other people consider life to have intrinsic value. They believe that just being born confers a basic worth and value on every human being. This value does not have to be earned; you are born with it. Basic human rights are the things everyone, including you, deserves simply by being alive. Among other things, you deserve to live, to have freedom of action, to speak. You deserve to have your needs met, to feel good about yourself, to respect yourself and have others treat you with respect. You deserve to feel safe, to choose whom to trust or not trust, to express yourself and to assert your other rights. These rights are not absolute; they have limitations. For example, no one has the right to harm another. These rights, and their limitations, are embodied in laws, the U.S. Bill of Rights, and other documents such as the United Nations Declaration of Human Rights. These institutions formally assert basic human value and worth because some people and nations do not hold these values. You may have encountered such a person who treated you as if you were worthless and without value. You do not, however, have to accept such a person's values. You have the right to choose your own. It is, after all, your life, not someone else's.

Others' values, of course, influence your own, and it is valid to decide that you agree with the values of others around you. What most matters is that you sort out and decide for yourself what is important. This is not always simple or easy. Much of what goes on around us is shaped by other people's decisions about what is and is not important. We often automatically accept these values without giving them much thought.

Money, Power, and Expectations

Money and power are common ways that people measure value in this society. It is easy to think of value only in these terms. For many people, money and power are important priorities; for some people they are *most* important. How important are these things to you? Why are they important? Do you sometimes measure your own and others' value in terms of money? What does it mean to you to earn more or less? What does it mean if others earn more or less? Despite the high value most people give to money, most would also agree that the value of a human life cannot be assessed with dollar signs. Human value relates to how we conduct our own lives and our place in the lives of others. This includes how we treat others and ourselves, our efforts to be kind, compassionate, honest, and respectful.

Power is another common way people gauge value. Presidents, prime ministers, and kings tend to be esteemed by virtue of their powerful positions. The reverse is also true; those with less power are often considered to have less value simply by virtue of their position. However, money or power cannot really confer value; they are valuable only to the extent they can be used to get you what you want or need and they have their limits. Money can buy many things but not self-esteem, trust, or intimacy. Basing your value solely or mostly on external things such as money makes your value fragile. A truly enduring sense of self-esteem is based on your internal sense of yourself and an appreciation of your whole range of attributes.

What qualities are important for you to have? What sort of person is it important for you to be? What do you expect of yourself when you expect the best? Answers to questions like these might help you see some of the values that you hold for yourself. You are probably most aware of your values when you fall short of them, but to evaluate yourself or others *only* on the basis of unmet goals is inaccurate and unfair. For example, people generally considered by others as successful often push themselves toward high goals. Yet those same people can think themselves failures if they don't completely live up to these high expectations. If you feel you are a failure, you need to ask yourself the three questions mentioned earlier:

- Who is doing the valuing? Can you separate what you really think from what others may think?
- What is the overall situation? Are you considering your own record over time or judging yourself by a single experience?
- What standards are being used? What is good enough? Might you be using the highest achievement as a measure of basic value?

It is unrealistic and even damaging to define value as perfection. Just as it is possible to feel safe enough with some risk, it is possible to feel worth, value, and self-esteem without being perfect. Human beings have limitations. You may sometimes fail because you try to do more than you can successfully handle. You might be more successful if you attempt fewer tasks. You may be accomplishing a great deal but *feel* stressed, uncomfortable, and a failure, because you are neglecting your own needs. When you neglect your own needs, it becomes harder and harder to do your best.

Even when you do your best, you will sometimes make mistakes. Mistakes are a normal, unavoidable part of everyday life. Mistakes do not mean total failure any more than perfection means value. When you begin to believe this, you will begin to feel much better about yourself.

WHAT DOES SELF-ESTEEM MEAN TO YOU?

You are a complex person with a variety of abilities, strengths, weaknesses, and gifts. Which characteristics do you feel most positively about?

What do you most like about yourself?

Why do you like this about yourself?

Do you have physical abilities that you feel good about? What are they?

What aspects of your body's physical appearance do you like?

Do you take care of your body? If so, how?

Do you have mental abilities that you like or enjoy? If so, what are they?

Do you like how you express emotion? What is it you like about that expression?

Do you take care of yourself emotionally? If so, how?

What do you enjoy doing for yourself?

Do you ever reward yourself? If so, when and how?

My five best qualities are

1. _____

2. _____

3. _____

4. _____

5. _____

Esteem for Your Self—Warts and All

Building a firm foundation of self-esteem means coming to terms with those parts of yourself you may not like but cannot change. Self-esteem does not require that you like every aspect of yourself. You may never be happy with how tall you are, or how serious you are. Having self-esteem means that, on the whole, you feel your value outweighs your shortcomings. In making this self-assessment, you need to be fair to yourself. You need to grant yourself basic human rights and you need to exclude those aspects of yourself over which you have no control, and for which you are not responsible. You have no control over how tall you are and you may have limited control over your basic temperament. You are stuck with these and probably other less-than-perfect attributes. But you can choose how important to you these unchangeable aspects of yourself are.

We ask you now to look at what you like *least* about yourself. This can be helpful when you see areas within yourself that you could change. But there may be things you don't like that you cannot change. Do you hold these things against yourself?

The five qualities about myself that I like least are

1._____

2._____

3._____

4._____

5._____

Could you realistically do anything to change any of the above? If so, what is it you could do? If you do not like these qualities but cannot change them, can you accept them as part of the whole package that is you? Can you allow them a place and still value yourself overall? If this seems very difficult to do, ask yourself why these qualities concern you so. Perhaps you are judging them according to other people's definitions of what is important.

Your Bill of Rights

You may never before have considered that you have personal rights, but you do. The following space gives you a chance to write a personal bill of rights. What do you think you have a right to expect from yourself and others? In the first section below, list the rights you are certain that you have. In the second section, list those things you wonder whether you have a right to. Perhaps you wish you had these other rights but you are uncertain if you actually do. We encourage you to find someone you trust in order to explore the second list and determine which items you might move up to the first list.

I have the right to . . .

_____

_____

_____

_____

_____

I wonder if I have the right to . . .

_____

_____

_____

_____

_____

SORTING OUT FACTS ABOUT ESTEEM FROM REACTIONS: SHADES OF GRAY

In Chapter 6 we explained that a real sense of control is based on knowing what you can and can't control. Self-esteem is based on knowing for what you can take credit and, just as important, knowing when it is unfair to hold something against yourself. Self-esteem is based on self-acceptance, which is feeling good about those things you do control and not punishing yourself for things you cannot. Self-acceptance and acceptance of others also play large roles in intimacy. We will discuss those more in the next chapter.

Exercise 7.1 (see page 242) offers a list of abilities that are important to appreciating your self-worth. How much or how little do you believe these abilities and qualities apply to you?

DO YOU HAVE ENOUGH SELF-ESTEEM?

Everyone makes mistakes; everyone also has value. Do you believe this about yourself? Do you like yourself? Do you believe you deserve to be treated with respect? Can you forgive yourself if you make a mistake? If your answer to these questions is "yes," you may have enough self-esteem. If it is "no," you may not value yourself as much as you need.

How did you rate the qualities and abilities in Exercise 7.1? It is possible to feel bad about yourself and yet agree that you have many of the abilities listed in Exercise 7.1. If this is the case, you may not fully realize the value of these various abilities. They are all important in helping you get what you need, in getting what you feel is important—whatever that may be. Perhaps you have been focused on what you cannot do and have forgotten many of the important things you can do. Reminding yourself often of these positive qualities will help give you a more balanced view of yourself.

EXERCISE 7.1 How Much Do You Know and Appreciate Yourself?

The following is a list of abilities that are important to appreciating your self-worth. Circle

1. I can almost always	4. Once in a while
2. Most of the time	5. Not often
3. Some of the time	6. Almost never

Quality	Almost always					Almost never
Know my feelings	1	2	3	4	5	6
Respect my feelings	1	2	3	4	5	6
Respect my own needs	1	2	3	4	5	6
Acquire what I need	1	2	3	4	5	6
Accept I'll make mistakes	1	2	3	4	5	6
Find ways to feel comforted	1	2	3	4	5	6
Know what is most important to me	1	2	3	4	5	6
Accomplish small goals	1	2	3	4	5	6
Reward myself for small accomplishments	1	2	3	4	5	6
Make mistakes and try again	1	2	3	4	5	6
Laugh at myself	1	2	3	4	5	6
Like myself	1	2	3	4	5	6
Feel a sense of personal value	1	2	3	4	5	6
Value another despite his/her failings	1	2	3	4	5	6
Feel loved, wanted, accepted	1	2	3	4	5	6

Time-Out for Self-Care: Affirmations for Self-Esteem

As you know by now, an affirmation is a positive statement you make about yourself or others. Affirmations can be important reminders of your own and another's value. An affirmation helps you refocus your attention away from your harsh internal critic toward your real abilities and strengths. An affirmation also reminds you that errors and mistakes are not the end of the world but a natural part of being human. They can coexist with self-esteem. You may repeat the following affirmations about control and esteem as often as you find helpful:

- I cannot control some things but I am not helpless.
- I cannot control other people but I am not helpless.
- I am not responsible for those things I cannot control.
- I accept those things in myself I cannot change.
- I can make positive choices for myself.
- My strengths and abilities deserve my appreciation.

Appreciate those abilities you have. Did you circle 1 or 2 for any abilities in Exercise 7.1? If so, those are true strengths. Remind yourself of them often. Create your own affirmations by completing the following sentences:

I am not powerless, I can _____

_____

I have the right to refuse _____

_____

I am not helpless, I can _____

_____

I deserve to _____

TRACKING REACTIONS TO BELIEFS ABOUT VALUE AND ESTEEM

Identifying Your Beliefs about Your Value

If you are uncomfortable with your current level of self-esteem, your beliefs about esteem and value could be getting in your way. Think now of a recent time when you felt low or bad about yourself. Use that specific situation to complete Exercise 7.2. See if you can identify a belief you have about your own value and worth. *Do not use a traumatic situation for this exercise.*

Maggie wanted to believe she was a valuable person; however, actually believing it was very difficult. She had been abused as a child and given the message that she was not deserving of respect. She tried forcing herself to feel valuable but willpower didn't work. She felt stuck. As she started to fill out Exercise 7.2, Maggie described the following situation:

I was treated as an object as a child and teenager.

Then she read the next question and asked herself, "What does this situation say or mean about me?" Then she wrote

Eventually, I came to believe that I am an object.

Then she had to ask herself, what does it mean to me that I believe I am an object. She wrote,

When I believe it, I act that way—like I'm not worth anything.

Then Maggie thought, what does it mean that I act as though I'm not worth anything?

I don't deserve respect from others and don't expect it.

This belief, based on her experience, is a powerful reason for Maggie's low self-esteem. As Maggie herself realizes, there are good reasons she came to believe she is not worth anything and does not deserve respect from others. This belief probably helped Maggie survive her years of abuse. The situation, however, is now different. Maggie is no longer a child. What does the belief do for her now?

Evaluating How a Belief Helps and Hinders You

Does Maggie's belief still help her now? If so, how much? How much does it get in her way now? Do the advantages of the belief outweigh the

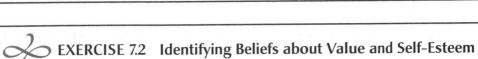

EXERCISE 7.2 Identifying Beliefs about Value and Self-Esteem

Think of a recent, everyday situation that led you to feel bad about yourself. *Do not use a traumatic situation for this exercise.* Describe the situation in the first blank below, then answer the first question. For each subsequent question, think mainly about what you wrote as an answer for the question immediately preceding it. If you have difficulty thinking of a situation, review your answers to Exercise 7.1. Did you circle 5 or 6 for any statement? Do those statements remind you of a recent situation?

Situation:

_____

_____

What does this say or mean about me?

_____

_____

_____

Looking at what I just wrote, what does *that* say or mean about me?

_____

_____

_____

What does *that*, in turn, say or mean about me?

_____

_____

_____

Looking at all the above, can I drawn any conclusions about myself?

_____

_____

_____

Adapted with permission from Dennis Greenberger and Christine Padesky, *Mind Over Mood: Change How You Feel by Changing the Way You Think.* New York: Guilford Press, 1995.

disadvantages? To find out, Maggie completed Exercise 7.3, which asked her to consider how the belief might help and hinder her. If you have identified a belief about self-esteem, fill out Exercise 7.3 now for that belief.

When Maggie answered the questions in Exercise 7.3, she realized some surprising things. For example, the belief that she was an object and deserved no respect was actually calming in a way. It helped her not get so upset when people treated her badly. Believing this about herself helped her feel that she, at least, understood herself. It certainly explained how other people had treated her and helped her make sense of the world. On the other hand, believing this also made her feel hopeless and helpless. If she really didn't deserve respect, then what hope did she have to feel better? There was also no point in even trying to get anyone's respect. Although the belief calmed her when bad things happened, that also meant she didn't fight much to protect herself. So the belief might not be so good for her in this way. The belief didn't help her make decisions because she thought she had no real choices. It also didn't help her know what she needed for herself. In fact, the belief made her think it was useless to bother thinking about that.

Pinpointing Problem Areas to Think Through Further

As a next step, review your answers to Exercise 7.1. For which abilities did you circle 4, 5, or 6? These may be abilities you do not yet have but can acquire. Do these tend to fall into one or more of the following general areas?

Knowing yourself

Valuing what *you* think is important

Acting on what *you* believe is important

Forgiving yourself for mistakes

Rewarding yourself for accomplishments

The five areas above condense some key abilities that contribute to self-esteem. Solid self-esteem is built on what *you* believe is of value when you consider yourself. You may, in fact, avoid considering yourself at all for fear that any imperfections mean you must be worthless. You may need to know yourself better and learn to recognize your strengths and not just your weaknesses.

EXERCISE 7.3   How Does This Belief Help and Hinder Me?

Most beliefs have both advantages and disadvantages. Consider those for the belief you identified in Exercise 7.2. Write down the belief in the space below, then circle how helpful or hindering the belief is for each question.

Belief: _____

Circle

1. Extremely helpful	4. Not at all helpful
2. Very helpful	5. Gets in my way
3. Moderately helpful	6. Gets in my way a lot

	Extremely helpful			Gets in my way a lot		
1. How helpful is this belief?	1	2	3	4	5	6
2. How calming is this belief?	1	2	3	4	5	6
3. How flexible is this belief?	1	2	3	4	5	6
4. How safe does this belief make me feel?	1	2	3	4	5	6
5. Does this belief help me understand myself?	1	2	3	4	5	6
6. Does this belief give me hope?	1	2	3	4	5	6
7. How essential is the belief to my survival?	1	2	3	4	5	6
8. How well does this belief help me cope?	1	2	3	4	5	6
9. Does the belief help me make sense of the world?	1	2	3	4	5	6
10. Does this belief help me make decisions?	1	2	3	4	5	6
11. Does this belief help me know what I need for myself?	1	2	3	4	5	6

Perhaps you know what is important to you, but you value what others think more. Why is this? Do you believe others are more deserving? Do you believe you have fewer rights? If this is the case, thinking through these beliefs may help you.

Do you have trouble accepting criticism and forgiving yourself for errors? Do you have trouble rewarding yourself when you accomplish even small things? If so, perhaps you believe that being of value can only mean something perfect or close to perfect. Perhaps your standards are unrealistically high. What alternative meanings might value have? What alternative standards of worth might be valid?

Taking Stock

All of this gave Maggie a great deal to think about. In fact, she felt a bit overwhelmed and wasn't sure what to do. Exercise 7.4 showed her what her choices were. She checked item 3. She did not want to think this through further right now. But she was beginning to see that there was more to think about whenever she felt ready to continue.

Take stock of how you feel right now. You may choose to stop now or continue thinking about self-esteem. Feel free to stop or take a break for self-care. Exercise 7.4 lists the options you have. Complete it as a record of where you are then move on to whatever you need to do for yourself right now.

THINKING THROUGH A BELIEF ABOUT VALUE AND SELF-ESTEEM

When you are ready, the exercises that follow help you look more closely at difficulties you may have with self-esteem. The next exercise asks you to think about a time when you have felt bad about yourself. Remember to take care of yourself as you answer these questions whether or not you believe you deserve such care. In fact, you do deserve it. Answering the questions in this book is difficult and you deserve to reward yourself as often as you feel you need.

EXERCISE 7.4 Taking Stock of Your Work on Self-Esteem

Consider what you think and feel right now. Do you wish take a break from this work? Do you wish to continue? Please check the statement that describes your situation right now.

_____ 1. My beliefs about my own value are fine. I do not need to think them through further. I am comfortable with the level of self-esteem I feel.

_____ 2. I am comfortable with how I value others. I do not need to think more about my beliefs on esteem for others.

_____ 3. I do not need to think through my beliefs about self-esteem right now although there are ways I do not feel comfortable. I can always come back at a later time if I want to think more about this.

_____ 4. I do not need to think through my beliefs about esteem for others right now although there are ways I do not feel comfortable. I can always come back at a later time if I want to think more about this.

_____ 5. I am beginning to think about why some of my beliefs about value and esteem do not work. I can continue thinking about this, but I want to move slowly and carefully. I can stop this work at any time.

_____ 6. I am ready to think through a belief about value and esteem.

If you checked 5 or 6 above, write down here any beliefs that you may wish to work on now or at some future time:

_____

_____

_____

_____

_____

_____

_____

_____

_____

_____

Choosing Beliefs to Work On

Make a list now of the beliefs you have identified so far that you would like to think through more carefully. Perhaps you have none, one, or several. Write down any that you have.

_____

_____

_____

For each belief you have noted, complete the questions in Exercise 7.5 (see pages 252–253). This exercise asks you to go over some of the same ground you have already thought about in earlier exercises, but then takes you a bit further. Select a belief, then think of a situation in which that belief influenced your experience. You can use the same situation you used to identify the belief in Exercise 7.2. Maggie came back to think further about her belief at a later point. Let's see how she filled out this exercise.

Sort Out the Facts of What Happened

At the end of Exercise 7.2, Maggie had written, "I don't deserve or expect respect from others." An incident had happened at work recently that left her feeling bad about herself. She decided to think through the belief using that situation.

Maggie worked as an administrative assistant for several managers. Different bosses gave her work, and she tried very hard to keep up with all of it. Then one day there was a crisis. One boss asked her to drop what she was doing to help him and she did. She stopped her other work, but a short time later another boss came around looking for his work. It wasn't done yet. He became angry and yelled at Maggie. This was the situation she described under the first question.

Sort Out the Meaning the Facts Have for You

The meaning of what happened seemed obvious to Maggie. She had been trying very hard to do a good job, but her efforts just weren't good enough. She had failed; she deserved to be yelled at.

Identify the Underlying Belief

The next question asked Maggie to take this meaning one step further. What was the larger lesson about herself that she saw in the experience? This too was very clear to Maggie. She wrote,

> I'm not good enough. I'm a failure. I don't deserve respect.

This was an old belief for Maggie. She had believed it for a long time, since her childhood experiences. Maggie realized the belief would not be easily or quickly changed. It could be changed but she needed to be patient. It would not change overnight.

Evaluate the Pros and Cons of the Belief

The next questions in the exercise asked Maggie to evaluate the belief. How did it make her feel about herself? How did it help her and how did it hold her back? When she thought of the belief she felt inadequate compared to other people. She supposed it helped her try harder, at least when it didn't make her feel hopeless. More and more, however, it did make her feel hopeless. However, it also helped her make sense of herself and of the world. Why else would people treat her that way? She must deserve it. She wished she had a better job but believed this was probably as good a job as she could get. She felt any better job might not be safely within her abilities. Now she wasn't so sure that she could even handle this job. The belief had held her back from trying for a better job, but perhaps that was a good thing because then, in her mind, she would only be a worse failure.

Imagine Alternative Meanings for the Same Facts

The next question asked Maggie to look again at the facts of what happened. What else could the situation have meant? This stumped her at first. She hadn't gotten her boss's work done. That was a fact. How could that not be a failure? To help her, she decided to reread earlier parts of this chapter and as she did that, she came across the three questions to ask yourself if you feel you're a failure. She asked herself these questions as she looked at the facts of what happened. The first question was

- Who is doing the valuing? Can you separate what you think from what others may think?

EXERCISE 7.5　Steps for Thinking Through a Belief about Valuing Self and Others

The belief you wish to think through:

_____

Sort Out the Facts of What Happened

Think of a particular situation in which this belief may have been a problem. You can use the same situation you used to identify the belief, or use another situation in which esteem or value was an issue. Describe the facts. What happened? What was the sequence of events?

Sort Out the Meaning the Facts Have for You

How did you interpret this situation? What did it mean to you?

Identify the Underlying Belief

What lesson did you draw from it about yourself? About other people?

When did you start believing this about yourself or others? Was this incident the first time? If not, when and how do you remember first learning this lesson?

Evaluate the Pros and Cons of the Belief

How does believing this make you feel about yourself or others? What does it make you think about yourself or others?

How does believing this help you or protect you?

How does believing this hold you back or get in your way?

Imagine Alternative Meanings for the Same Facts

Look back at your description of what happened (the first question above). Are there other ways to interpret what happened? What else could the situation mean? Is there an alternative meaning that would fit the facts of what happened? If so, what is it?

Evaluate the Pros and Cons of the Alternative Meaning

What positive feelings do you have when you think about this alternative meaning?

What negative feelings do you have when you think about this alternative meaning?

Consider How to Check the Accuracy of These Beliefs

How could you test to see whether or not your belief is true?

How high is the risk if you test the truth of what you believe? How dangerous would it be?

What good things might happen if you test the truth of what you believe?

Put the Process in Perspective

Will testing the belief matter 10 years from now? Would it help or hinder you in the future?

At first, this question didn't seem relevant at all. When it comes to a job, Maggie thought, what the boss thinks *is* what's important. It could mean keeping your job or losing it. On the other hand, Maggie had more than one boss. At least the boss whom she had helped during his crisis was still happy with her. She wasn't a failure in his eyes. The other, unhappy boss seemed to matter more. Why? Maggie thought it was her job to keep all the bosses happy, but she realized that each boss thought his own job was the most important.

- What is the overall situation? Are you considering your own record over time or are you judging yourself by a single experience?

When Maggie thought about this question, she realized that she was usually able to handle the workload. A few times in the past, she'd been a little behind, but she'd managed to get the work done before anyone started yelling at her. Actually, she hadn't been all that much behind this time either. What was different was the way she had been yelled at. She must have really messed up or he would never have yelled at her like that. His yelling filled her with shame.

- What standards are being used? What is good enough? Might you be using the highest achievement as a measure of basic value?

Maggie felt that she was doing a good job if she could keep all the bosses happy. She also saw that each boss wanted his own work done and didn't pay much attention to what else she had to do. Was she being fair to herself? Maggie remembered a section earlier in the chapter about being fair to yourself. It said, "You need to grant yourself basic human rights and you need to exclude those aspects of yourself over which you have no control, and for which you are not responsible." Maggie slowly realized that she did not have control over how much work she had to do. Actually, nobody did. Each boss gave her his own work without paying attention to how much she had from the other bosses. Each one acted as if he were the only one giving her work. Nobody was really keeping track. Actually, she hadn't been keeping track either. She'd been swamped but figured they knew what they were doing. Now, she wasn't so sure about that. What was the right thing to do if two bosses both had important jobs at the same time? Maybe it was impossible to keep all the bosses happy all the time. Perhaps one alternative interpretation was that she'd been doing a good enough job in a bad situation. Perhaps the boss who yelled at her was being unfair.

Evaluate the Pros and Cons of the Alternative Meaning

Maggie felt a flash of anger at her bosses when she first thought of this alternative meaning—but then she felt fear. She could see herself complaining about the workload; they would say she just couldn't cut it. Was she a failure or was the workload difficult for anybody to handle? Her usual response would be to just try harder but that was what she was already doing and look what happened.

Consider How to Check the Accuracy of the Belief

Maggie wondered whether another person would also have trouble in her job. That made her wonder about the person she was hired to replace. How had that person handled the workload? Maybe that was something she could ask one of her coworkers.

Put the Process in Perspective

Maggie still believed that she had failed and the shame she felt was hard to bear. She even started thinking she might quit the job. But if she was ready to quit the job over this, then maybe there wasn't a lot more to lose by asking a few low-risk questions. If it wasn't her fault, then she would feel so much better.

Time Out for Self-Care

When Maggie finished Exercise 7.5, she felt exhausted. She wanted to check out her belief by asking a few very low-risk questions—but not right away. When you finish Exercise 7.5, you may also want to take a break from this work. You do not need to move forward right away. You may want to take time to reward yourself at this point. This is difficult work and you deserve to care for yourself.

WEIGHING THE EVIDENCE ON BELIEFS ABOUT VALUE AND ESTEEM

Brainstorm Ideas for Collecting Evidence

When you feel ready to check the accuracy of a belief on value or esteem, the next step is to generate lots of low-risk ideas for doing this. Brainstorming is the method we recommend. You can use Exercise 7.6 or a blank piece of paper.

We do not want you to do anything high risk, but if high-risk ideas are in the front of your mind, you might get them out of the way by writing them down and then moving on to other ideas. Be sure to brainstorm ways for checking the alternative interpretation as well as the old belief. Some ways to gather evidence will work for both but some may not. To help you, we again list the categories of low-risk ways to check the accuracy of a belief.

1. Notice or observe specific events or actions and the people acting.

2. Watch other people's reactions to the event or action.

3. Notice when you yourself are already carrying out actions that produce evidence about your belief.

4. Ask friends questions about their reactions.

5. When it feels safe enough, take a small action with a safe friend and see how the friend reacts to you.

Watching and observing did not seem to fit Maggie's situation well. Asking her coworkers seemed the best strategy, but she needed to think carefully about whom and what to ask. She could imagine someone telling her that the incident was her own fault and she just didn't work up to standard. She wanted to keep her risk of this happening as low as possible. She thought of the person in the office with whom she felt most comfortable. Then she thought of possible questions. She felt nervous just thinking about any conversation along these lines and so she decided to plan out how this one conversation might go with this coworker. As she thought about this, she was automatically considering the risk.

**EXERCISE 7.6   Brainstorm Ideas for Collecting Evidence
on a Belief**

Create a list of rough ideas for collecting evidence on a belief. The goal is to come up
with some low-risk ways to collect evidence, but be prepared that the first ideas you
have may be high risk. Write them down to get them out of the way. You do not need
to carry out *any* of the ideas you write down. You will screen these ideas later and discard any you choose. Begin by writing down a belief and an alternative interpretation
on which you want to collect evidence. In the blank space below, write down any and
all ideas that come to mind for how to do this.

Belief: _____

Alternative interpretation: _____

Rank Ideas by Lowest Risk First

One idea was to invite her coworker Kim out to lunch. They'd be away from the office and maybe it would be a little less risky there. She could ask if Kim remembered the last person who'd held Maggie's job. Had she done a good job? Were the bosses happy with her? Had things worked the same way they do now with several people giving work to the one assistant? None of these questions was directly about Maggie. It was about the past, before Maggie had taken the job.

Depending on how Kim responded, Maggie could either drop the subject, or else ask other questions. If Kim seemed sympathetic and friendly, maybe Maggie could say something like, "I guess everybody heard me being yelled at the other day." Depending on how Kim responded, Maggie could decide to drop the subject at this point. If Kim seemed safe enough, Maggie wanted to ask what Kim thought she could have done to avoid the incident.

If you are considering collecting evidence about a belief, rank your own ideas by risk, lowest risk first. You can use Exercise 7.7.

Carry Out Lowest Risk Ways to Collect Evidence

After Maggie thought up this plan, she felt nervous about it. She couldn't do it right away but that was fine. She respected how she felt and waited. She took a week or so just to watch Kim and the other people around the office. She wanted to think more about how safe a person Kim seemed to be for the sort of conversation she had planned. She noticed some things during this time that she had not noticed before. Right after she had been yelled at, she had felt so ashamed that she had avoided much interaction with the others in the office. Now that she was paying attention to her coworkers, she noticed that a few of them occasionally made fun of the bosses behind their backs, especially the one who had yelled at her. He didn't seem to be liked much by the others. Meanwhile, several people did considerate things for her. Kim, in particular, had seemed very friendly lately, which is why Maggie thought she might be safe to talk to.

Maggie finally did ask Kim out to lunch and asked her first question about the person who'd held the job before her. To Maggie's surprise, Kim jumped right in sympathizing with Maggie over the hard time the one manager had given her. And also saying how surprised she was Maggie hadn't

EXERCISE 7.7   Baby Steps for Testing a Belief about Valuing Yourself and Others

In the first blanks below, write down the belief you are thinking of testing and an alternative interpretation. When you have brainstormed ideas for possible ways to collect evidence on a belief, rank those ideas by risk, starting with the lowest risk ways. List only ways that are within a reasonable risk. *Do not list any high-risk ways to collect evidence.*

Belief: _____

Alternative interpretation: _____

Least Feared Actions/Observations

_____

_____

_____

_____

_____

_____

_____

_____

Most Feared Actions/Observations

complained about it. Kim clearly thought Maggie had a right to complain. It turned out the company had had trouble keeping someone in that position, because of the way the job was organized. Other people had had trouble too. In fact, Kim told Maggie she was the best one they'd had so far in that job.

Clearly there were problems with Maggie's job, but she now had some evidence that the problems were not all her fault. It helped her feel much better and helped her look at the existing problems in a new way. She decided to keep watching for evidence and to record and weigh that evidence over time.

Record and Weigh the Evidence for and against the Belief

If you have a belief you want to continue testing, keep a running log of the evidence and then weigh the evidence. You can use Exercise 7.8 and 7.9 (see pages 261 and 262) to do this. Be sure to gather evidence on *both* an existing belief and an alternative meaning. Doing this will make the exercises much more useful to you.

SUMMARIZING YOUR WORK ON VALUE AND SELF-ESTEEM

Consider now what you need for yourself. You can put this workbook aside for now or you can continue to work on it as you choose. You may move on to the next chapter on intimacy or you can revisit part of this or earlier chapters. Feel free to identify other beliefs about value and esteem, evaluate them, and test how accurate they may be. When you are ready to stop your work on value and esteem, fill out Exercise 7.10 (see page 263) as a summary of your work. Review this summary when you come back. It will give you a sense of where you are and what else you might want to work on.

By virtue of being alive, you have value and you deserve respect, from yourself as well as from others. This is a right, not a reward. You cannot lose your basic human value when you make errors and mistakes, even when the consequences are terrible. It is our nature as humans to be imperfect and make mistakes, and yet we all still have basic worth. You can feel ashamed of imperfections and still have value. It is only fair that you grant yourself the same basic human worth and respect that most of us in this society grant to each other. To value yourself is to know and appreciate who you are—warts and all.

EXERCISE 7.8   What Evidence Do I Have about the Existing Belief?

What evidence do you already have about the accuracy of your existing belief? What facts, words, or actions support the belief? What facts, words, or actions indicate the belief is inaccurate? Write those down below.

Belief: _____

What facts or evidence support this belief as accurate?

1. _____

2. _____

3. _____

What facts or evidence indicate this belief is not accurate?

1. _____

2. _____

3. _____

How sure are you that this belief is accurate? Mark how sure on the following scale. Use the second evaluation scale later to check on changes in your beliefs in light of new evidence.

Date: _____

Accurate   Inaccurate

_____

100%   50%   0%

Date: _____

Accurate   Inaccurate

_____

100%   50%   0%

**EXERCISE 7.9   What Evidence Do I Have
about the Alternative Meaning?**

What evidence do you already have about the accuracy of the alternative meaning?
What facts, words, or actions support the alternative meaning? What facts, words, or
actions indicate the alternative meaning is inaccurate? Write those down below.

Alternative meaning: _____

What facts or evidence support this interpretation as accurate?

1. _____

2. _____

3. _____

What facts or evidence indicate this interpretation is not accurate?

1. _____

2. _____

3. _____

How sure are you that this interpretation is accurate? Mark how sure on the following
scale. Use the second evaluation scale later to check on changes in your beliefs in light
of new evidence.

Date: _____

Accurate   Inaccurate

_____

100%   50%   0%

Date: _____

Accurate   Inaccurate

_____

100%   50%   0%

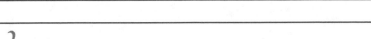

EXERCISE 7.10   Summarizing Your Work on Value and Self-Esteem

I have identified the following beliefs about valuing myself and others:

I can think of the following alternative meanings:

I have carried out the following steps (mark with X); or I would like in the future to carry out the following steps (mark with *):

_____   Make a list of what evidence might confirm and/or contradict the existing belief.

_____   Organize the list of evidence from least feared/least risky to collect to most feared/most risky to collect.

_____   Carry out the least feared/least risky way to collect evidence.

_____   Keep a record of the evidence collected—both pro and con.

List here any evidence collected—what did you see or do, and how did it turn out? Continue adding to this list over time, as you become aware of additional evidence.

CHAPTER EIGHT

Feeling Close to Others

YOUR NEED FOR INTIMACY: The need to know and accept your own feelings
and thoughts; the need to be known and accepted by others.

INTIMACY is a difficult art.

> —Virginia Woolf, "Geraldine and Jane,"
> *The Second Common Reader*

HOW INTIMACY CAN BE AN ISSUE AFTER TRAUMA

We all need to feel in touch with ourselves and to connect emotionally with others. This connection, whether with yourself or another, is based both on how well you *know* and how well you *accept* the different parts of yourself. But trauma changes you. What you thought you knew about yourself may also have changed. There may be aspects of yourself that you are experiencing for the first time and so they feel strange or unfamiliar. When this happens your sense of intimacy with yourself, and with others, can be disrupted or destroyed.

Feeling a Stranger to Yourself

The powerful mix of feelings experienced during and after a trauma may be unlike anything you have ever felt before. If you do not know how to identify your feelings, you may experience them as alien, without reason, or as something to get rid of. If we asked, "How do you feel?" you might respond, "I don't feel anything," or "I don't know." You may not know why you cry, don't cry, rage, or withdraw. The ways you feel and act may not make sense to you. In these ways trauma can make you feel as a stranger to yourself.

> ✿ *Sylvie's relationships tended to be explosive and unpredictable. After several failed marriages, she found herself on the brink of moving in with a man she was dating. Within days of the moving date, Sylvie became upset with her boyfriend and a tremendous scene resulted. He wound up taking away her copy of his house key, and she moved her possessions out of his house. However, unlike other times, Sylvie realized that she had been ignoring feelings of fear and anxiety about moving in with this man until they burst out in a fight. When she thought about it, Sylvie saw that making this type of commitment in the past had always been the beginning of the end of a relationship. In this light, her feelings began to make more sense. Once Sylvie admitted her true feelings to herself, she could make a better informed choice about how to handle the move and her relationship.*

Survivors of trauma often cut themselves off from feelings or try to ignore them, as Sylvie did. It's a way to protect themselves from feeling overwhelmed. It is possible to go through life numbed, thereby avoiding some of life's pain. However, the costs of doing this are high. Cutting off feelings can put you at greater risk. Feelings, both good and bad, provide crucial information to help you take care of yourself and your relationships. Buried feelings tend to show themselves one way or another, such as through stress-related illness or sudden eruptions of tears, rage, or grief. Life's spontaneous pleasurable feelings may also be cut off along with painful feelings. It may be tempting to seek short cuts to comfort, through excessive alcohol or other drug use, food, sex, or work—but these behaviors can become addictions. You may feel you need them so you don't feel panic, anxiety, depression, emptiness, fear, or other states. Yet these feelings are all aspects of yourself. Knowing yourself means listening to the messages that these feelings bring you. It is the experience of learning to tolerate and work through these feelings gradually, at your own pace, that brings healing and relief.

Feeling Disconnected from Others

Intimacy with others is based on how much you allow others to know you. But there is always risk in doing this, because we cannot control how others will respond to us. The ability to intimately connect with others is therefore affected by your sense of safety, trust, control, and self-esteem. Disruptions in these other needs can disrupt your abilities for intimacy.

❧ *Robert grew up in a violent home. His father was an alcoholic and often beat the members of the family. Robert's mother, brothers, and sisters each coped in his or her own way, not relying on anyone else in or outside the family. Robert became an expert at survival. However, he never learned to be in a close relationship in which he could rely on another person and share his true thoughts and feelings. As an adult, he continued feeling separate and estranged from others.*

Intimacy can also be disrupted by the traumatic loss of someone with whom you have grown deeply connected. The death of a spouse, child, parent, sibling, combat buddy, close friend, or other important person in your life can be a traumatic break in your human connection, not just with that person, but with anyone. The pain of loss can be so great that the risk of any connection can outweigh the hope. You may be afraid to love again, or to allow yourself deep feelings for another. You may protect yourself by allowing others to get only so close and no closer. You may end relationships as soon as the beginning stage passes and closeness deepens. Ending relationships on a conflicted or negative note can become a pattern. Although self-protective in some ways, isolation can leave you feeling dissatisfied and lonely. It can also reinforce a belief that intimacy with others is impossible, but this belief is not necessarily true.

Trauma Survivors Speak about Intimacy

• I needed people to listen to me tell my story, sometimes over and over. Lots of the people in my life disappointed me and added to my losses. New people entered my life and cared for me and listened. Five years later, I am still walking alone much of the time and I long for more connections. Finally now I know I can find the community I seek and I feel more patient about the process of growth; it's like waiting for spring flowers to rise from the snow and waiting for them to bloom.

• Intimacy is something I am very afraid of. It's something I don't trust and I am not sure I am going to be able to.

• Intimacy is being able to share feelings and thoughts with another person. Intimacy is being there, daring to know, sharing the good and bad. Intimacy is mutual and means resolving problems between two people. Intimacy is powerful, magical love, trust; it is reciprocal honesty and safety; it is closeness and togetherness.

Various phases of healing are likely to occur over time, even over a number of years. You may, for example, feel a wave of grief or other emotions when you reach the age your parent was when he or she died. Even after reaching a comfortable sense of peace and healing, you will probably continue to process your experience in various ways for a long time. Written many years following the sudden death of the author's father, the following poem reflects a continued connection with a cherished person in the face of loss. While her father died during her childhood, she continues to reflect upon and learn about her relationship and connection with her father, and the impact of his death upon her.

The Stillness of Trees
The trees you planted
when "just a wee lad"
stand there
still
keeping the promise you
forgot.

They reach toward a sky
streaked with stratus clouds—
the same sky whose stars we
charted and mapped,
marking seasons and time.

You said trees tell stories
if we care to listen.
Ear to bark and branch
we'd stand,
hearing their tales
like leaves whispering
upon wind.
I feel a voice

now
in the stillness of the trees.
But these pines
no longer speak to me
since sky splintered
and fell.

Sharing scarlet sunsets
no longer
you lie so still
in suit and tie.
You must be sleeping,
I think,
touching your cheek
as I pass.

Later,
I place pine cones—
Sugar and Digger
(our favorite)
at your feet.

Your promise
of returning,
of always,
and forever
standing
still
as the oak
by which you
sleep.

                        Katherine L. Heenan

WHAT CAN INTIMACY MEAN?

When we think about intimacy, we think of emotional warmth, closeness, caring, and support from and with other people. An intimate relationship is, almost by definition, a safe and trusting relationship in which each person values and cares about the other. But as we've tried to show, safety, trust, and esteem can each mean different things to different people in different situations. The meaning of intimacy for you will depend to a great extent on what these other needs mean and how much of each you need. However, intimacy is also something we all need in its own right.

We all want to be valued and accepted by another, to be emotionally connected to another for our real selves, our deepest thoughts and feelings. But some people believe this isn't possible, or possible only at a high price. Do you think you have to give up something important in order to be close to another person? Do you think you must choose between being selfish but alone, or selfless but with someone? If so, you may be seeing intimacy in all or nothing terms. Neither is an attractive choice and fortunately, these are not the only choices. The psychologist Harriet Lerner, in her book *The Dance of Intimacy,* sees intimacy as a process of navigating connectedness with another. It does not have to mean giving up the separateness that is your self. In fact, intimacy is most possible when each person knows and values his or her own self. As Lerner puts it,

> An intimate relationship is one where neither party silences, sacrifices, or betrays the self and each party expresses strength, vulnerability, weakness and competence in a balanced way. (p. 3)

The essence of what *you* need from intimacy is to be known and accepted for who you really are—your real self with all its quirks and imperfections. This is always a risky process because you cannot control other people's reactions to you. Not everyone will, in fact, accept you as you really are. Because intimacy involves the risk of rejection, you need to be able to protect yourself until you feel the risk is acceptable and worth taking. Although we cannot control others' reactions to us, we usually can control how much we reveal of ourselves. This is one way to take care of yourself in relationships.

The smooth functioning of society depends on people controlling many of their immediate impulses and not fully revealing everything about themselves to whomever comes along. This is good. Most of us go through our day-to-day lives wearing a socially acceptable mask. We put our best foot forward. We don't advertise our mistakes. We do this because we want people to think well of us, to accept us. Our efforts can work; people often do accept us but only as far as we've let them know us. Our social mask often hides large parts of who we really are. Intimacy, however, is about letting another peek behind the socially acceptable mask. Until we've begun to do this—and it need not be done all at once—we haven't really given ourselves an opportunity for intimacy.

Intimacy is most often earned and strengthened gradually through a mutual interaction with another person. Like trust, it is earned. It can be thought of as a process of sometimes small actions, small risks, by one person followed by responses and sometimes small risks, from the other. The process can then loop back, building on what's gone before. When successful, the process of building mutual intimacy has two basic steps: (1) letting another know you, followed by (2) the other accepting you. You control the first step including what, when, and how much you reveal about yourself. You do not control the second step, being accepted. However, it can be easy to miss or mistake another's acceptance when you get it. It is important to be able to recognize acceptance when you see it. An important part of developing intimacy with another person involves your accepting him or her. Similarly, a feeling of closeness with yourself is fostered by self-acceptance.

The Risk of Letting Yourself Be Known

The foundation of intimacy with another is in knowing yourself. We have encouraged you to know yourself better throughout this workbook. Knowing yourself can be difficult because it involves knowing things you may not like or want to acknowledge—not only your strengths but also your weaknesses; not only your joys but also your doubts and fears. The possibilities for intimacy with another are shaped by the following:

Knowing and trusting what you *feel and think* about things

Knowing what feels, and is, *safe* enough for you

Knowing when and how much to *trust* another

Knowing what is important to you and *valuing* yourself enough to express it

Knowing what you can and can't *control* about yourself and other people

Knowing what you can accept about the other person

How much or how little of each need is truly acceptable to you? What level of risk is acceptable in seeking intimacy? It can be difficult to hold on to yourself in a relationship when you do not know who you are and what you need. Only you can know what you feel and need. Real intimacy can grow only when you get enough of your other needs met. Expressing those needs is part of your power in a relationship. Expressing yourself—who you are, what you need, revealing yourself—is a part of the process most in your control. If you don't feel safe or trusting enough with the other person, perhaps for good reason, this will impede the process. If you don't value yourself enough, this will impede the process. If you don't understand what you can and can't control in the relationship, that too can impede the process.

You cannot control how another person responds to you. True intimacy requires that person's free and honest response. This is why an accepting response is a valuable gift. But what is an accepting response? When you like another person but don't like what he or she has just told you, how do you respond? Do you feel you have to offer acceptance or lose the friendship? What does acceptance really mean?

Being Accepted; Accepting Another

The essence of acceptance is nonjudgment. This is the core of what we need from intimacy. However, acceptance, like intimacy itself, is not all or nothing. Rather, it is a reaction to who you are as a whole person. It is possible for people to accept you as a person, but dislike specific individual traits you might have. Perhaps you are a smoker. It is possible to have good friends who accept you but find smoking unacceptable. If you and your friends value each other enough, there are probably ways to accommodate both of you. You may choose to go without smoking much of the time, whereas your friends might not object to your smoking with them outdoors. Each individual needs to decide for him or herself what problems can be overlooked or accommodated, and which might be truly unacceptable. Most of the time, this is not an all or nothing, like-it or lump-it sort of choice.

Acceptance can be confused with powerlessness, resignation, and with having no real choice. This is not how we mean it. All-or-nothing choices are generally unacceptable. For example, if being safe means zero risk and intimacy always involves risk, then you must give up one need. This is *unacceptable*. You need both. The only truly *acceptable* choice is one that allows you to get enough of both. Being able to accept something means that overall, it is *enough* of what you need. The same principle holds when the needs of two separate people seem to conflict. Both people need safety, trust, esteem, control, and emotional intimacy. As long as neither person believes these needs are all-or-nothing, each is likely to define what they need in somewhat different ways and to somewhat different degrees.

We all need acceptance despite our imperfections but how do you know when another accepts you? What signals do you look for? How do you signal your own acceptance to another person? This can vary from person to person. There are, however, some signals that are frequently understood to mean acceptance. For example, acceptance and intimacy are often signaled by closeness. Lack of intimacy or acceptance can be signaled by distance. The physically closer we are to someone, the more we can physically sense and know about him or her. We can see, hear, smell, or touch the other person; he or she can do the same with us. We think of touch as the most intimate of our senses because it requires us to be closest. But a person close enough to touch is close enough to hurt. This is why there is always some risk with intimacy, just as there is with trust. Intimacy requires us to trust that those we allow close to us will not intentionally harm us. True intimacy is caring and supportive but people are imperfect and so is intimacy. Even the best intentions can go wrong. Without wanting to, people who are intimate can and do hurt each other. Intimate relationships can survive unintentional hurts because knowing each other deeply means knowing that each is imperfect. This makes it possible to forgive.

Because we think of intimacy as being close, our sexual relationships are often considered our most intimate. Giving birth, nursing, being born, and having sex are the physically closest that people come to each other. Ideally, such physical closeness is an extension of emotional closeness, but the two are not necessarily the same. It is possible to have one without the other. People healing from sexual or physical abuse can develop emotionally intimate relationships but sometimes need extra time before feeling safe with sexual contact. People often develop emotionally intimate relationships with their psychotherapists but it is unethical for the therapist to engage in a physical relationship with a client. At the same time, a sexual relationship can lack emotionally intimacy. Having sex will not, by itself, create emotional intimacy that is otherwise lacking in a relationship.

What then can closeness mean when we are talking about emotional intimacy? Some people think it means sameness. Being as much like the other person as possible is a kind of closeness. One way of trying to be accepted is by belonging. Similarities and belonging can be part of emotional connection but they do not guarantee it, nor do differences block it.

Some people think intimacy means agreeing or at least not disagreeing with the other person. Yet because people are different from each other, differences are bound to happen. Intimacy does not require that individuals give up their own opinions, preferences, and desires when they differ from the other person's. Some people think that intimacy cannot coexist with conflict or disagreement but fortunately, this does not have to be the case.

Other people think intimacy means wanting to be together all the time, or as much as possible. Spending time together is a way people can get to know each other and become emotionally close. Physical nearness isn't required for emotional connection, however. Intimate emotional connections can be made and maintained over long distances through letters, the telephone, or over the Internet. This is possible because intimacy grows out of knowledge about another and of the other about you. This can happen naturally, and sometimes quickly when we share important emotional experiences with others. A trauma such as a natural disaster can be such an experience—emotionally connecting people on the basis of their shared knowledge of the experience. If you have difficulty reconnecting with your close friends and family after the trauma, it may be because they don't have the personal knowledge of the experience that you have. Other trauma survivors may be more likely to have that knowledge. This is why joining a support group of survivors is one way to begin to reconnect and find intimacy again.

Shared intense experiences can create strong emotional bonds between people but intensity is not the same as intimacy. The strength of feelings waxes and wanes. Intimacy is better measured by the depth of knowledge people have about each other. How strongly someone cares about us is actually less important than that they continue to care about us as they know us better and better over time. Being known deeply, however, does not mean that everything about yourself must be revealed. Emotional closeness can coexist with areas of personal privacy.

Intimacy is not sameness *or* difference, closeness *or* distance, physical nearness *or* physical separation, complete knowledge *or* personal privacy, agreement *or* conflict. Rather, intimacy exists between each of these things; it is always some mix of all of them.

Sameness, nearness, intensity of feeling, time spent together, agreement, lack of conflict, and sex can all be signs of acceptance but none is essential. What is essential to acceptance is nonjudgment. Without the other person's basic acceptance of who you really are, the relationship will not meet your needs for intimacy. Acceptance means that the other person still values you, despite knowing your flaws and imperfections. True acceptance means that the other person will not try to change you—not only because they know they can't but also because they value you.

Intimacy doesn't happen overnight. Knowing someone well, being able to trust his or her response, and accurately reading that response are all ingredients of learned and earned intimacy. New intimacies begin with two people who may not know each other very well. But it can be difficult to correctly read another's response unless you already know the person well. How does the other person "read" you? How do you "read" them? Do you really know what's going on? When someone learns something new about us will they still stay as close or will they back away? Will the tone of their voice stay as warm or get a little cool? These can be subtle signals, and it is not always easy to read them correctly. For example, what does another's silence mean to you after you have made some personal disclosure? Do you assume that it means acceptance and the other person is waiting for you to continue and tell more? Or do you assume it means distance and the other person does not really approve and doesn't want to encourage you to continue. Among other possible meanings, silence can sometimes mean either of these things. Intimacy can shrink or grow depending on how you interpret others' responses to you. Your beliefs about yourself and others will shape what you think other people mean. Your interpretations may or may not be accurate.

Accepting Differences

Similarities increase the likelihood that people will accept you—at least for those things you share with them. Similarities reduce the risk of revealing yourself. It's easier to express support of the local sports teams at home games than at away games. Even with similarities, however, people have differences. Will other people accept you when they begin to see the ways you are different from them? Do you ever give others a chance to see? Can you be who you are when that means revealing the ways you are different, unique, or imperfect? True intimacy doesn't have a chance until you begin to risk finding the answers to these questions.

Do you have difficulty accepting other people who are different from you? Do you expect others to reject you when you are different? If so, you may think that sameness means acceptance and approval, whereas difference means disapproval. You may have trouble accepting the differences in others if you interpret them as criticisms or rejections of the way you are. Differences usually have nothing to do with judgments. People cannot always control the ways in which they are similar to or different from others. When they can, choosing to be different is often a way to express a unique self. Choosing something different does not have to be a judgment about others.

> ❀ *Ted and Darryl found out they were both avid basketball fans. They started going to games together and had a good time. Ted always bought and ate hot dogs during the game but Darryl never wanted one. During one game, Darryl mentioned that he was vegetarian and didn't eat meat. Ted immediately thought the comment meant that he did not approve of Ted's hot dog. Ted got irritated and said, "What do you want me to do? Throw it away?" But this isn't what Darryl meant at all. Darryl simply wanted to tell Ted something important about himself. He hoped that Ted could still accept him once he knew about this difference.*

Ted is not likely to accept Darryl's vegetarianism if that means Ted has to give up hot dogs around Darryl. If Darryl tries to correct the misunderstanding, perhaps Ted will be able to accept this difference. Whether or not Ted accepts this difference in Darryl depends on many different things. This includes how the conversation goes from this point. Will they just get angry and cut each other off or will they try to understand what each really means? If they have enjoyed their friendship up until this point, this difference isn't likely to jeopardize their continued friendship.

WHAT DOES INTIMACY MEAN TO YOU?

Intimacy with other people develops from knowing yourself and what you need. How well are you getting to know yourself as you go through this workbook?

Do you know when to check in and listen to your own thoughts and feelings? Can you notice when you are beginning to feel sad, numb or upset?

How do you respond to your needs and feelings? Do you

____ try to ignore them?

____ listen but put them off as less important than other things?

____ take them seriously and try to act on them if that is what's needed?

Have you ever stopped to care for or comfort yourself while reading this book? At other times?

Each of the following is a way to build a greater intimacy with yourself. Have you tried any of the following? If you haven't, which of them do you think might help you?

____ Write in a journal

____ Talk to someone who has been through something similar to what I went through

____ Read books about my experiences

____ Pay attention to my feelings and try not to judge myself for having those feelings

____ Listen to my own ideas without judging them

____ Slow the pace of my life so that I have time to notice my feelings and reactions

____ Take time to check in with myself by asking, How do I feel about this? What is going on in my body as I think about this? What do I need in this situation?

____ Make plans to allow myself time to relax and reflect (for example, take a bath, walk outside in nature, read poetry, meditate).

____ Remain drug and alcohol free

____ Spend time with friends

____ Turn to friends for support when I need someone to talk to

____ Use touch in appropriate, healthy ways without violating others' boundaries, such as asking for hugs from safe others when I need them

____ Use my personal things to soothe myself: wear a favorite piece of clothing or jewelry, carry a favorite stone

Thinking back over your life, what has been your closest relationship? Even if that relationship has ended, think now about the qualities that made it emotionally intimate. With whom did you have this intimate relationship?

What qualities of this person, or your interactions with him or her, made you feel close and intimate?

What did this person know about you that felt personal and intimate (e.g., thoughts, dreams, feelings, interests, doubts, fears, etc.)?

Did you feel accepted? If so, what made you believe this person accepted you?

What did you know about this person that felt personal and intimate (e.g., thoughts, feelings, doubt, fears, interests, etc.)?

Did you accept the person *in spite of* knowing these things? Did you accept the person *because* you knew these things?

How did you show you accepted the person?

It is very possible to be deeply known and accepted emotionally, and not be physically or sexually intimate. The reverse is also true, but physical intimacy without emotional intimacy can feel, and be, risky. Intimacy is closeness, but *close* can mean different things, in different situations, to different people. Think about meanings of closeness when answering the following questions.

How do you let others know you care about them?

How do others let you know they care about you?

How do you define the word *love?*

What types of love have you known (for parents? siblings? friends? children? romance? etc.)?

What types of love can you give safely?

SORTING OUT FACTS ABOUT INTIMACY FROM REACTIONS: SHADES OF GRAY

All of your relationships exist on a continuum between care of yourself and care for others. Intimacy does not mean that you or the other person must give up your basic needs in order to have the relationship. But you must know what needs are more and less important to you. Intimacy requires not only a thoughtful negotiation with yourself so that you can balance your own various needs, but it also requires a thoughtful negotiation with another person to balance his or her needs with your own.

Intimacy can vary and grow depending on *what* you disclose about yourself and to *whom*. What specific types of information about yourself do you consider personal, intimate, and revealing of who you are? How well do you already know the other person? Both considerations are important when you decide whether or not to risk further closeness. How risky does it feel to disclose this information to an acquaintance, a friend, or the person closest to you? Exercise 8.1 asks you to consider different kinds of information that you may or may not consider as personal or intimate. Information that you feel is high risk to disclose about yourself may or may not seem intimate to another. One person might find it very difficult or risky to reveal passionate interests to another person, whereas another finds that not very risky at all. Some people have trouble admitting any worries or problems, others feel boastful when talking about something going well. Fill out Exercise 8.1 (see pages 282–283) to begin considering what information you feel is high risk to disclose to another, and which is low risk.

Although the essence of acceptance is nonjudgment, people show each other acceptance in different ways and to different degrees. Acceptance can look different in different relationships. Regardless of how emotionally close you now feel to your parents, you probably still have an intimate emotional connection that dates to childhood. You might also have a close friend who is an important support and confidante, as well as a lover or spouse with whom you have an emotionally and physically close relationship. Each of these relationships will be different; you may look for and expect somewhat different things from each one. They can all meet the basic need for intimacy as long as you feel these people know you deeply and accept you enough.

There is no way that acceptance, love, and emotional caring can be proven with certainty. However, you may feel that it is not safe to reveal your deepest self unless others prove themselves in some particular way.

> ❦ *Amy's best friend is Charlotte. She has grown to depend on Charlotte for friendship and emotional support. But she can't shake the fear that Charlotte will one day decide to drop her as a friend. Part of Amy doesn't believe that anyone can really like her once they get to know her. However, Amy also wants to feel safety and trust in their friendship so she keeps wanting Charlotte to prove it to her. One day they had a disagreement. Amy said that if Charlotte truly cared for her, she would do what Amy wanted. Charlotte did truly care for Amy, and she was willing to talk over some things, but agreeing with Amy meant giving up care and control over herself. This she didn't want to do.*

If Amy could control Charlotte's behavior—which she cannot—it might make her think she was safer, at least for a little while. But even that couldn't prove Charlotte's friendship was totally safe and trustworthy. There is no *proof*, but there is *evidence* of Charlotte's acceptance and caring. The evidence is her continued presence as a friend, even in the face of Amy's unreasonable demand. Amy's fear that Charlotte might leave distracts her from seeing that Charlotte is actually still there.

It is important to be able to recognize acceptance when you see it. Acceptance is not all or nothing. It is not about the other person giving up one of her needs—say for control—so you can have one of yours—say safety.

♾ EXERCISE 8.1 Weighing the Risks of Revealing Different Aspects of Yourself

Intimacy requires that you let yourself be known. But some aspects of yourself are riskier to disclose than others. This exercise asks you to consider the kinds of information you feel most comfortable and least comfortable sharing in a variety of circumstances. For each category of information, such as your passionate interests, give a specific example then rate that specific piece of information.

How risky to disclose	Least risky				Most risky	

1. Your passionate interests

Example: _____

How risky to disclose						
to an acquaintance	1	2	3	4	5	6
to a friend	1	2	3	4	5	6
to the person closest to you	1	2	3	4	5	6

2. Important things about you that are similar to the other person

Example: _____

How risky to disclose						
to an acquaintance	1	2	3	4	5	6
to a friend	1	2	3	4	5	6
to the person closest to you	1	2	3	4	5	6

3. Important things about you that are different from the other person

Example: _____

How risky to disclose						
to an acquaintance	1	2	3	4	5	6
to a friend	1	2	3	4	5	6
to the person closest to you	1	2	3	4	5	6

4. What you most value about yourself

Example: _____

(continued)

How risky to disclose						
to an acquaintance	1	2	3	4	5	6
to a friend	1	2	3	4	5	6
to the person closest to you	1	2	3	4	5	6

5. Details of a bad day when you made mistakes or were blamed for problems

Example: _____

How risky to disclose						
to an acquaintance	1	2	3	4	5	6
to a friend	1	2	3	4	5	6
to the person closest to you	1	2	3	4	5	6

6. Asking for help with a personal problem

Example: _____

How risky to disclose						
to an acquaintance	1	2	3	4	5	6
to a friend	1	2	3	4	5	6
to the person closest to you	1	2	3	4	5	6

7. Letting the person know when he or she is doing something that bothers you

Example: _____

How risky to disclose						
to an acquaintance	1	2	3	4	5	6
to a friend	1	2	3	4	5	6
to the person closest to you	1	2	3	4	5	6

8. Asking a person to explain what they meant when they said or did something

Example: _____

How risky to disclose						
to an acquaintance	1	2	3	4	5	6
to a friend	1	2	3	4	5	6
to the person closest to you	1	2	3	4	5	6

Rather, acceptance is about talking and thoughtfully negotiating about how each of you can get enough of what you both need. What Amy most needs is something that Charlotte cannot give her: self-acceptance. But Charlotte's friendship can help Amy move toward that if she doesn't have to give up her own sense of value and self-control.

What does acceptance look like? By what signs might you recognize it? The next section will help you figure this out.

How Well Are You Known and Accepted?

An intimate relationship usually requires the mutual cooperation and effort of both people. It is a process of give and take. You can give by revealing parts of yourself. You can give by listening to and learning about someone else. In giving, you may gain many things for yourself but giving alone will not meet your basic needs for intimacy. For that, you need to be on the receiving end. What you need are people who listen to you and accept you. If you are doing all the listening and accepting, if the relationship is all give but no take on your part, then you are probably not getting your intimacy needs met.

Exercise 8.2 describes aspects of an intimate relationship from the receiving end only. Complete Exercise 8.2 now and rate how accurately each of the statements describes your experiences in your closest intimate relationships. Consider your emotionally closest friends and remember that sexual relationships are not automatically the emotionally closest ones. A psychotherapy relationship can be one of your most emotionally intimate. It is a special kind of relationship that is more one-sided than most others. It focuses on your emotional needs and not those of the therapist. A good therapist meets his or her own emotional needs in other relationships. This is why it can be easier to feel known and accepted in psychotherapy than in other relationships. If you wish, you can think of your therapist as you fill out Exercise 8.2. Whether you are thinking of a close friend, partner, or your therapist, when you get to the physical intimacy question, think in terms of how physically safe and comfortable you feel just being around that person. Perhaps not touching is what is most safe and respectful to you right now. When you finish, read the next section to find what your answers might mean.

EXERCISE 8.2   How Well Are You Known and Accepted for Who You Are?

The statements below describe ways that another person in a relationship gets to know you and shows that he or she accepts you. The statements below cover only the other person's role in an intimate relationship. Think of a relationship that you felt was intimate. How well were you known and accepted in that relationship? Read the statements, then circle the number that matches your experience in that relationship.

Circle

1. Always	4. Sometimes
2. Most of the time	5. Rarely
3. Often	6. Never

	Always					Never
He/she makes time to be with me without distractions.	1	2	3	4	5	6
Even though it's sometimes difficult, he/she listens to how I feel.	1	2	3	4	5	6
He/she respects my need to spend some time alone.	1	2	3	4	5	6
He/she respects my need to spend some time without him/her but with other people.	1	2	3	4	5	6
He/she can enjoy being with me without alcohol or other drugs.	1	2	3	4	5	6
I am able to enjoy physical intimacy with her/him in a manner that feels safe and respectful to me.	1	2	3	4	5	6
He/she generally tries not to control my feelings.	1	2	3	4	5	6

(continued)

❦ EXERCISE 8.2 (continued)

Circle

1. Always   4. Sometimes
2. Most of the time   5. Rarely
3. Often   6. Never

	Always					Never
He/she generally tries not to control my actions.	1	2	3	4	5	6
He/she enjoys our common interests but also respects our differences.	1	2	3	4	5	6
I have fun with him/her.	1	2	3	4	5	6
I feel safe letting my guard down with him/her.	1	2	3	4	5	6
I trust that he/she will not intentionally harm or humiliate me.	1	2	3	4	5	6
He/she respects growth and change in me.	1	2	3	4	5	6
I feel supported by him/her.	1	2	3	4	5	6
He/she stands by me in good times and difficult times.	1	2	3	4	5	6

ARE YOU GETTING ENOUGH OF WHAT YOU NEED FROM INTIMACY?

As we said in Chapter 3, everyone needs a minimum level of intimacy with other people. Specifically, this means, you need to be *known and accepted for who you really are.* This does not mean that everyone needs to accept you. This is impossible. Most of us need only a few people to know and accept us.

Being accepted does not mean being liked for your every quality or for every thing you do. You only need to be accepted, overall, as a whole. Being accepted means that the other person values and cares about you enough to accept or forgive your flaws, imperfections, or annoying traits.

Reread the statements down the left side of Exercise 8.2. Have you ever experienced the kind of relationship described in these statements? Were you able to circle "often" for many of the statements? If so, you probably know how it feels to get what you need in an intimate relationship. Are you in such a relationship now? If yes, you have an important intimate support and you may not need to work further on intimacy. Sometimes, even when you have a single intimate connection, you may wish for additional close relationships. Relying solely on one relationship for closeness can put great pressure on that relationship. You might feel lost or disconnected when that person is not available. If so, then you may not be getting enough of the emotional intimacy and support that you need.

In the space below, list the people with whom you feel emotionally closest. Are they family members? spouse? friends? therapist? Write in the names. Then, for each person, ask yourself if your sense of closeness has changed since your traumatic experience. In the space to the left of each name write whether you feel closer, more distant, or the same degree of closeness now as you did before. If your trauma occurred in childhood, you may or may not be able to complete this portion of the exercise. Still, list the people with whom you are closest as a guage of some of the support you have.

Has Your Closeness with Others Changed Since the Trauma?

People close to you: *Closer? The same? More distant?*

_____   _____

_____   _____

_____   _____

_____   _____

If you can list several people and your relationships have remained close since before your trauma, this is good. Your trauma experience may not have affected your abilities for intimacy. You can probably get the support you need. Some relationships may even have grown closer since the trauma. As you risk talking to people about yourself and the changes you have experienced they will know you even better. By talking about how you really feel and think, you give others the chance to accept you as you are now, changed or not. Feeling accepted in this way is a mark of true intimacy.

If any of your relationships have grown more distant since the trauma there could be many reasons. For starters, the problem in connecting may not be with you but with others. It is good to be able to talk about your experience with someone supportive. But perhaps those closest to you cannot bear to listen to what happened in the way you need. This is understandable. The more someone cares about you, the more upsetting he or she may find your trauma experience. This is no one's fault, but it may mean you need to look elsewhere, at least for a little while, for the support you need. Joining a support group of trauma survivors or talking to a counselor or therapist may be helpful if this is your situation.

Problems with intimacy can occur when you believe intimacy means only one thing, or must mean something completely. When intimacy proves imperfect, as it always does, you may believe that it has been destroyed and cannot be recovered—but this is not the case. You may be mistaking intimacy for just one of the ways in which it can be signaled. You may not be recognizing all the various forms that intimacy and acceptance can take. If you think you may have a problem with intimacy, the next section will help you begin to figure out where the problems might lie.

BALANCING INTIMACY WITH OTHER NEEDS

Intimacy must be balanced with the other needs discussed in this book: safety, trust, self-esteem, and control. The ongoing task of every relationship is finding and maintaining the middle ground where both people get enough of these basic needs met. Neither person will be able to have these needs completely and totally filled. But each should be able to have enough, as each defines enough.

Intimacy runs into trouble when you think it means either you *or* the other person, not both, can have their needs met. You have basic needs; the other person has basic needs. What happens when those come into conflict? Do you have to choose between the other person or yourself having your needs met? How can you balance valuing yourself and what you need with valuing another person and what they need? Exercise 8.3 (see page 290) will help you address these questions. Think again of a relationship you consider emotionally close, or think of a relationship you wished were more intimate. Then rate how well each of your needs were met during that relationship.

As you complete the exercise for yourself, you may want to read how Ruth filled it out. She used her relationship with her current boyfriend, Jim. She feels very close to him and wants the relationship to be good for her. You may feel this way too as you do this exercise. But it's important to be as honest with yourself as you can.

Intimacy and Safety in a Relationship

The first question in Exercise 8.4 tested how honest Ruth was going to be with herself. It asked how safe she was with Jim. Her immediate thought was that, of course, she was safe. On second thought, she admitted he had a temper, and he had hit her sometimes. She didn't like this but he was always so sorry afterward, she felt sure that he really cared for her. This question, however, doesn't ask about what Jim thinks or feels. It asks only what Ruth thinks or feels about her own need for physical and emotional safety. As we have mentioned, the need for safety is

- the need to feel that you are reasonably protected from harm inflicted by yourself, by others, or by the environment, and
- the need to feel that people you value are reasonably protected from harm inflicted by yourself or others

Another way to think about this is to ask if you have ever felt frightened in the relationship—whether for yourself, for the other person, or by the other person. The truth is that Ruth had felt a bit scared. She decided to circle 4. It was on the danger side of the scale but not far along it.

Ruth had grown up in a family in which her parents hit the kids frequently. Wasn't that how they showed they cared? Although Ruth has rea-

∞ EXERCISE 8.3 How Well Can You Meet Your Other Needs in an Intimate Relationship?

Think of a person to whom you feel emotionally close. With that person and relationship in mind, read the following questions, and answer by circling the number that best corresponds to your answer.

How physically safe are you with this person?

Totally safe _____ In great danger

1	2	3	4	5	6

How emotionally safe are you with this person?

Totally safe _____ In great danger

1	2	3	4	5	6

How much do you trust and depend on this person?

Total trust_____ Total disappointment

1	2	3	4	5	6

How much control and power do you have in the relationship?

Complete control _____ Powerlessness

1	2	3	4	5	6

How much do you value your own needs and feelings in the relationship?

Completely _____ Not at all

1	2	3	4	5	6

How emotionally close do you feel to this person?

Extremely close _____ Extremely distant

1	2	3	4	5	6

sons for believing that hitting is a sign of caring, it is not. She is confusing care with control. Parents often need to restrict or limit their children's choices in order to keep them safe and to teach them basic skills. True caring and acceptance are about respecting other people, whether children or adults. Hitting is disrespectful. Regardless of what it is for, hitting another person is *always unacceptable*. No one has the right to be violent toward another. If you are hit in any relationship, or threatened physically, you are in a degree of danger in the relationship.

Intimacy and Trust

Next Ruth thinks about her own needs to trust. As we discussed in Chapter 5, there are two aspects of this need. Specifically

- the need to rely on your own judgment, and
- the need to rely on others to meet some of your needs

These two aspects of trust are often mixed together in an intimate relationship. For Ruth, having Jim as her boyfriend means she has already made a judgment about him. She has a stake in the relationship's working out to show that her judgment was sound. However, judgments are based on the specifics of a situation and those specifics can change. Ruth's judgment about Jim can and should shift as she gets to know him better and has more information about him. For example, Ruth has evidence that Jim can be thoughtful and considerate. He was a big help when her car broke down. On the other hand, last week he canceled out on her for a date at the last minute and that makes her more unsure of him than she was before. He said he had an unexpected emergency but he was vague about it. She doesn't know if she believes him or not. Earlier she might have circled 2, but now, she decides to circle 3 on the trust versus disappointment scale.

Intimacy, Power, and Control

The next question asks you to consider issues of power and control in an intimate relationship. Recall that your needs for power and control are

- the need to control your own actions and to express what you think and feel, and
- the need to have some effect or influence on others in your life and in your environment

Just being able to attract Jim as a boyfriend makes Ruth feel powerful. But she wonders if she can hold on to him. When she thinks just about the balance of power in the relationship, Ruth feels that Jim holds all the cards. She wants him to like her. So she really goes out of her way to do what he wants. His temper also encourages her not to cross him. She circles 4 on the control versus powerlessness scale.

Intimacy and Self-Esteem

This question asks you to weigh how much you valued yourself in the relationship. If you and the other person disagreed, did you feel you had as much right to your opinion as the other person? Or did he or she somehow count more or count less? Did you consider his or her feelings, needs, and wants as more or less important than your own? Did you value yourself enough to express what you really thought, felt, and needed, even if it was different from the other person?

Ruth felt good about herself because she had attracted Jim, but she didn't feel that good about herself otherwise. In fact this was one reason it was so important to her to hold on to Jim as a boyfriend. If he stuck around, didn't that mean she was worth something? She couldn't really decide what to circle on this scale. She felt in the middle and so she put a circle halfway between 3 and 4 on the scale.

How Well Do You Balance Intimacy with Other Needs?

Take a look at your own answers for Exercise 8.3. Can you get your other needs met in a relationship? Did you circle 4, 5, or 6 for one or more of these needs? If so, you may not be getting enough of that need met. If you also circled 1 or 2 for at least one other, you may be trading off one basic need to meet another. In some relationships, perhaps you feel comfortably safe but not very close or perhaps you feel very close but powerless. Perhaps your relationship is high in trust and closeness but low in self-esteem or power. If your relationships are high in closeness, but low in some other need, ask yourself if you believe intimacy means giving up that other need. Do you think that valuing yourself highly means you cannot be close to another? Do you think that being in control of your feelings, actions, and choices means you cannot be close to another? If the answer is "yes" to any of these questions, you may be thinking of intimacy or another need in all-or-nothing terms. Of all the needs covered in this workbook, however, intimacy is the one that most requires you to let go of all-or-nothing thinking.

Look at how you answered the last five statements in Exercise 8.2. These statements are about feeling safe, trusting, respected, supported, and having someone to depend on. If you circled 1, 2, or 3, you almost certainly have an emotional connection with this person. The lower the number, the deeper and stronger the connection. This is good; however, it may or may not be enough intimacy for you. Even when you have single, intense emotional connection, such as with a spouse, you can still have unmet needs for emotional connection. Your spouse or partner may not be able to give you emotional connection and support in all areas. Being emotionally connected to a range of friends, at varying levels of closeness, may be what you need.

Time Out for Self-Care

If completing the exercises so far has overwhelmed or upset you in any way, take time out to care for yourself. Talk to others or try the relaxation exercises found elsewhere in this book. Staying in touch with what you want and need for yourself is a basic building block for intimacy with others.

TRACKING REACTIONS TO BELIEFS ABOUT INTIMACY

As mentioned above, if you are struggling in the area of intimacy, the problem may be with your own beliefs about intimacy, with the other person, with the interaction process between the two of you, or some combination of all three. How can you tell? It can help to look at the interaction process first. Your reactions to another person depend on what you think his or her actions or words mean. There can be a gap between what you interpret and what that other person really means. Other people may also misinterpret what you mean. Sometimes the problem is simply a matter of not saying clearly enough what is meant. Sometimes the problem is more complicated. The following section is designed to help you sort out the facts of an interaction— what was done and said—from what was meant. If a belief about intimacy is part of the problem, that may show itself as you look at the interaction process.

Sorting Out Facts from Meanings: Examining the Interaction Process

When you interact with anyone, but particularly with lovers, close friends, or relatives, the interaction process can either help build intimacy or hinder it. Both people participate in the interaction, and there are several points at which the process can go astray. Understanding the steps in the process helps pinpoint where there might be a problem. Specifically, here is what happens:

1. You listen to your own feelings and thoughts to know what you need or want.
2. You act (or choose not to act) to express what you need or want.
3. The other person interprets the meaning of your action/nonaction.
4. The other person responds based on what he or she thinks your action/nonaction means.
5. You interpret the other's response based on what you think he or she means.

Let's look at an example of this sequence in action. This process can describe a casual chat with a coworker about a TV show, or it can describe an intimate conversation with a partner or relative. When we are talking with someone close to us, we are more likely to assume that we know what he or she means. This is often a safe assumption. When people are close, we know them better, but we can never know another perfectly. Misunderstandings happen even with the closest friends. Let's look at an example of the interaction process in action.

❀ *Yvonne came home from work stressed and overwhelmed after a chaotic day. She was very quiet and withdrawn. Her husband didn't notice, didn't ask what was wrong, and didn't do anything to help her feel better. He went about his business. Yvonne felt he must not really care about her.*

We can break down the above incident into the five steps as follows:

1. Yvonne hears her own feelings and thoughts. She feels stressed out, upset, and overwhelmed.
2. Yvonne acts by becoming very quiet and withdrawn.
3. Yvonne assumes that her husband interprets this action correctly.

4. Yvonne assumes that her husband responds to her message by going about his own business.

5. Yvonne assumes his response means a lack of concern for her.

Yvonne could be right that her husband is not concerned for her—but she could also be wrong. Yvonne is assuming a number of things in the interaction that may or may not be accurate. Exercise 8.4 offers a list of questions to help you analyze your interactions. Yvonne used these to figure out what might be going on between her and her husband. The exercise starts by asking you to think of a recent situation where you either failed to make an emotional connection when you wanted to or a connection broke when you didn't want it to. In the situation space, at the start of the exercise Yvonne wrote:

I came home from work upset, and my husband didn't even notice or care.

Then she looked at each question in turn. Here's what she wrote as she answered.

1. *Did you know how you felt, and what you wanted for yourself?*
Yvonne knew the answer to this.

I felt overwhelmed and upset. I wanted comfort.

It is important to have a sense of what you are feeling and want from the other person in an intimate situation, but we don't always know this. Sometimes, it is only after a disappointment—when we don't get what we want—that we clearly realize what we do want from the other. When this happens, you have a choice about what to do next. You could just give up and believe you have blown your chance, or you could see that you now have a second chance to ask more clearly for what you want. It is not in anyone's power to read our minds, not even those closest to us. However, it is in Yvonne's power to know her own mind and then ask for what she wants or needs.

2. *Did you let the other person know how you felt and what you wanted? How?*
Yvonne first wrote, "yes," because she thought she had shown husband how she felt and what she wanted from him. Then she thought about how she had shown him. She did what she always did, she got very quiet and withdrew into herself. This was how people in her family behaved when they got

EXERCISE 8.4   Examining the Interaction Process

Think of a recent situation in which you either failed to make an emotional connection when you wanted to or a connection broke down when you didn't want it to. Describe the facts of the situation in the space provided, then answer the following questions about it.

Describe the facts of the situation:

1. Did you know how you felt, and what you wanted for yourself? If yes, what did you feel and want?

2. Did you let the other person know how you felt and what you wanted? If yes, what did you do to let the other person know?

3. Did the person correctly understand the message you sent? How do you know?

4. Describe as objectively as possible what the other person actually said or did in response.

5. What do you think this response meant?

6. Is there another way to interpret this response? What else might it have meant?

upset. Growing up, she had learned that it wasn't always a good thing to ask directly for comfort or help. Her parents expected the kids to be independent, strong, and handle most things on their own. When she did ask for help or emotional comfort, she was often told she shouldn't be so upset. Asking for help in her family seemed to mean you were weak and couldn't handle something on your own. It was shameful to ask for help. But everybody needs help sometimes, even the people in her family. When they really needed comfort or help, they would get quiet and withdrawn. It was a signal her family understood. It was a way of asking without asking. But her husband had not grown up in her family. Did he understand what the signal meant?

3. *Did the person correctly understand the message you sent? How do you know?*
The message of Yvonne's upset was so clear to her that she assumed her husband must have gotten it. He must know her well enough to know what it meant when she withdrew. But did he? She couldn't remember that they had talked about this pattern. She finally had to admit she wasn't sure if he really understood what she meant or not.

4. *Describe as objectively as possible what the other person actually said or did in response.*
Yvonne wrote, "My husband did not seem to notice anything wrong with me. He did not ask me what was wrong. He did not offer any help."

5. *What do you think this response meant?*
Yvonne wrote, "He doesn't care about me. He can't handle it when I'm having a difficult time. He wants me to feel good and be strong all the time." Yvonne could be right about the meaning of this response. The odds of her being right would increase if the message had come from her parents or siblings. She could also be wrong about what her husband meant. The odds of her being wrong increase because her husband did not grow up in her same family.

6. *Is there another way to interpret this response? What else might it have meant?*
Yvonne was able to come up with two alternative meanings. She didn't quite know whether to believe either one, but had to admit each was possible.

1. Maybe he knows something is wrong and is just giving me some space. Maybe he's not sure how to comfort me.

2. Maybe he really doesn't notice anything is wrong. It's not fair to expect him to read my mind. Maybe he had a hard day himself and is distracted by that.

Yvonne learned at least one thing from this exercise. She expected her husband to know when she needed comfort without her asking for it directly. Part of her felt that he shouldn't "make" her ask because that felt so shameful. On the other hand, how could she really expect him to read her mind? In some ways, knowing another's mind was part of what intimacy meant to her. She felt she was good at anticipating her husband's needs, doing things for him before he had to ask, but he didn't seem to do the same for her. Yvonne thinks that her husband could at least try to anticipate her needs. He doesn't seem to even try.

Yvonne has discovered areas in which the basic communication process may have gone astray. Maybe she could be more clear and direct about what she needs and wants. Making an effort to do so could be all that's needed. But the situation feels more complicated to Yvonne.

Identifying Beliefs about Intimacy

The exercise on examining the interaction process helps you sort out the facts of a situation from what you think those facts mean. Yvonne's hurt and angry reactions to what happened are based on her interpretation that her husband doesn't really care about her. This exercise won't necessarily help you identify a core belief about intimacy, but it could. Yvonne saw that she believed that a large part of intimacy was being able to anticipate the other person's needs and wants.

You may or may not have already identified a core belief about intimacy. If you haven't, try to identify a belief now by filling out Exercise 8.5. Once again start with a situation in which you wanted to make an emotional connection but didn't or else an emotional connection broke down when you didn't want it to. *Remember, do not use a traumatic situation for this exercise.* If you wish, you can use the same situation you used earlier for Exercise 8.4.

EXERCISE 8.5   Identifying Beliefs about Intimacy

Think of a specific situation in which you felt a problem emotionally connecting with someone. This could be a situation in which you felt the other person failed to know you well enough or failed to accept you in some way. *Do not use a traumatic experience for this exercise.* Describe the situation, then answer the first question below. For each following question, think about your answer for the question immediately above it.

Situation:

_____

_____

What does this say or mean about me?

_____

_____

Looking at what I just wrote, what does that say or mean about me?

_____

_____

What does that, in turn, say or mean about me?

_____

_____

Looking at all the above, can I drawn any conclusions about me?

_____

_____

Adapted with permission from Dennis Greenberger and Christine Padesky, *Mind Over Mood: Change How You Feel by Changing the Way You Think.* New York: Guilford Press, 1995.

It may also be useful to pinpoint where your difficulties with intimacy might lie. If you are dissatisfied with the level of emotional closeness in your relationships, consider whether you might have all-or-nothing beliefs about intimacy. The following qualities, in moderation can be part of an intimate relationship. None of them, however, is required for intimacy. We have stated most of these qualities in an extreme form. Do you believe that an intimate relationship *must* have one or more of these qualities?

- Being the same, being as much like each other as possible (e.g., race, ethnicity, religion, education, tastes in food, entertainment, values, where to vacation, etc.)
- Being physically together, spending every available free moment with each other
- Having a sexual relationship
- Having complete knowledge of the other person, no secrets between you
- Being in complete agreement
- Never arguing, never being in conflict
- Believing you will never be hurt in the relationship
- Believing the other person will take care of all your needs
- Always feeling intense caring or other positive emotions
- Knowing what each other wants without asking

Do you believe that being close and intimate with another means the two of you cannot disagree? Do you feel intimacy requires a sexual relationship? Do you believe that the other person must be willing to take care of all your needs or else they don't really care? If you agree with these above statements, you may have all-or-nothing beliefs about intimacy in that area. As you read through this chapter are you reminded of a particular situation or incident? If so, use that situation to fill out Exercise 8.5. Yvonne had already identified a belief about intimacy from the earlier exercises. She moved directly on to Exercise 8.6 which helped her evaluate how the belief helped and hindered her.

Evaluating How a Belief Helps and Hinders You

Yvonne believed that intimacy meant the other person would know what she needed or wanted without her asking, and vice versa. She now evaluated that belief by filling out Exercise 8.6 (see page 302). Yvonne's belief about intimacy had both advantages and disadvantages for her. For example, when her husband did figure out how she felt and what she needed, she felt taken care of, calmed, and very safe and secure. But the belief did not help her know what she needed for herself. It made her depend on someone else for what she wanted or needed. She was beginning to see that the belief was very disempowering. But she was afraid that if she were more direct about her needs, her husband would back off and she'd lose the intimate relationship. That fear may have been somewhat accurate when she was a child, but how accurate is it in her relationship with her husband? Maybe she could speak more openly and freely about her needs with him without risking their intimacy.

How do you rate your belief about intimacy? Does it help more than hinder? Could this belief be hindering you more than helping? If so, you might want to think further about it either now, or at a later time.

IMAGINING, AND EVALUATING, AN ALTERNATIVE INTERPRETATION

When Yvonne examined the interaction process with her husband, she was asked to think of an alternative meaning for her husband's response. She thought of three alternative explanations:

1. He knows something is wrong but is giving me space.
2. Maybe he doesn't know how to comfort me.
3. Maybe he really doesn't notice anything is wrong with me.

When Yvonne considered any of these alternative interpretations, she felt hopeful—but there was also anger mixed in with the hope. She very much wanted to believe that her husband did care about her, but even if one of the above interpretations were right, perhaps her husband might not give her what she needed. Her fears about this may be right, but they could also be wrong. She hasn't tried to actually check out what may or may not be accurate.

EXERCISE 8.6   How Does This Belief Help and Hinder Me?

Most beliefs have both advantages and disadvantages. Consider those for the belief
you identified in Exercise 8.5. Write down the belief in the space below, then circle how
helpful or hindering the belief is for each question.

Belief: _____

Circle

1. Extremely helpful	4. Not at all helpful
2. Very helpful	5. Gets in my way
3. Moderately helpful	6. Gets in my way a lot

	Extremely helpful					Gets in my way a lot
1. How helpful is this belief?	1	2	3	4	5	6
2. How calming is this belief?	1	2	3	4	5	6
3. How flexible is this belief?	1	2	3	4	5	6
4. How safe does this belief make me feel?	1	2	3	4	5	6
5. Does this belief help me understand myself?	1	2	3	4	5	6
6. Does this belief give me hope?	1	2	3	4	5	6
7. How essential is the belief to my survival?	1	2	3	4	5	6
8. How well does this belief help me cope?	1	2	3	4	5	6
9. Does the belief help me make sense of the world?	1	2	3	4	5	6
10. Does this belief help me make decisions?	1	2	3	4	5	6
11. Does this belief help me know what I need for myself?	1	2	3	4	5	6

Taking Stock

Pause now to consider what you need and want. Do you want to continue working on intimacy? Do you want to put this work aside for now? Feel free to stop now if you choose. If you prefer to work on other issues right now, feel free to do so. Exercise 8.7 (see page 304) asks you to take stock of where you are in your work on intimacy. Fill this out as a record, then move on to do whatever you need to do right now. If you checked items 5 or 6, then continue on in this chapter by reading the next section.

WEIGHING THE EVIDENCE

The best way to check out what another person means is to talk it over with the other person. This is particularly important, but it can also be difficult in intimate relationships. When a close friend or partner misreads you, it reveals that there are limits to how well he or she knows you. Coming up against these limits can hurt. It helps soothe the hurt to realize that there are inevitably going to be limits to how well we know anyone; all of us are human and imperfect. In fact, after you know someone well, it is often through misunderstandings that you learn what it is you don't yet know about each other. Talking over these hurts and misunderstandings with the other person is the best way that you both get to know and accept each other better. Intimacy is strengthened and deepened by talking over those times when intimacy fails.

When Yvonne was ready, she considered how to check out her interpretations of the incident with her husband. In considering baby steps to check out your beliefs about intimacy, you may find it easy to think of questions but you also need to consider *how* to ask the question so that you really are keeping an open mind.

Yvonne still felt angry and this was a problem. As with collecting evidence on other needs, it is very important to keep an open mind. Her anger indicated that Yvonne might not be as open minded as she needed to be. For example, Yvonne could talk to her husband about why he didn't respond to her being withdrawn, but if she speaks angrily, blaming him, she isn't keeping an open mind. Her husband is much more likely to respond with his own anger than giving her any real information. She could, however, tell him she

EXERCISE 8.7 Taking Stock of Your Work on Intimacy

Consider what you think and feel right now. Do you wish to take a break from this work? Do you wish to continue? Please check the statements that describe your situation right now.

_____ 1. I am comfortable with the level of connection and acceptance I have with myself. I do not need to think more about intimacy and myself.

_____ 2. I am comfortable with the levels of intimacy that I have with other people. I do not need to think more about intimacy and other people.

_____ 3. There are ways that I might not have enough of a connection and acceptance with myself, but I do not wish to think more about this now. I can come back to this whenever I feel ready.

_____ 4. There are ways that I might not have enough intimacy with others, but I do not want to think more about this right now. I can come back to this issue whenever I feel ready.

_____ 5. I am beginning to think about why some of my beliefs about intimacy do not work well. I can continue working on this, but I want to move slowly and carefully. I can stop this work at any time.

_____ 6. I am ready to think through a belief about intimacy with myself or others.

If you checked 5 or 6 above, write down here any beliefs that you may wish to work on further now or at some future time:

_____

_____

_____

_____

_____

_____

_____

_____

_____

_____

feels hurt and explain why she feels hurt. She could tell him that, for her, intimacy means knowing what the other wants without being asked. She could ask if her husband shares this belief. If he doesn't, that too could explain his behavior. If this is not a signal of intimacy to him, then what is? How, then, does her husband show he cares? Could he be giving signals that he cares that she doesn't recognize? When Yvonne did sit down to talk about this, she was able to tell him why she was hurt, in spite of still being a little angry. Her husband turns out to have been distracted by his own day at work and had not noticed Yvonne's quiet withdrawal. He told her to ask when she needed comfort or attention from him. She told him it was very important that he try sometimes to see what she needed without her asking. As they talked further, she began to realize that maybe it was unfair to make him read her mind; but he also began to see that he wasn't doing much else to let her know that he, in fact, did care.

Yvonne and her husband already had a close intimate relationship that enabled them to resolve their problem more quickly. Let's look at another relationship at a much earlier stage of intimacy.

> ❄ *Long after being abused as a child, Ellen still experienced great shame. As an adult, she never spoke with anyone about her traumatic experiences and no one knew of the ways she fought flashbacks, high levels of anxiety, and almost constant fear. She believed that letting anyone close to her would result, at best, in harsh judgment and humiliation. She had caring friends, but kept them at arm's length even when they expressed concern about her. After much thought, she decided to risk revealing herself a little more. She planned to tell her closest friend a few pieces of her story. If the friend seemed to listen and still accept her, Ellen could decide to reveal a little more about herself. This could be done through a series of small self-disclosures over a long period of time.*

Ellen carefully thought out what she might reveal about herself and how risky or safe each piece of information felt to her. She used the brainstorming Exercise 8.8 (see page 306) to keep a record of her ideas even though the process wasn't all that quick.

It took her a long time to accumulate a number of things she might reveal that felt low risk enough. When she had a number of ideas, she ranked those items lowest risk first, on Exercise 8.9 (see page 307).

EXERCISE 8.8   Brainstorm Ideas for Collecting Evidence on a Belief

Create a list of rough ideas for collecting evidence on a belief. The goal is to come up with some low-risk ways to collect evidence, but be prepared that the first ideas you have may be high risk. Write them down to get them out of the way. You do not need to carry out *any* of the ideas you write down. You will screen these ideas later and discard any you choose. Begin by writing down a belief and an alternative interpretation on which you want to collect evidence. In the blank space below write down any and all ideas that come to mind for how to do this.

Belief: _____

Alternative interpretation: _____

EXERCISE 8.9   Baby Steps for Testing a Belief about Intimacy

In the first blanks below, write down the belief you are thinking of testing and an alternative interpretation. When you have brainstormed ideas for possible ways to collect evidence on a belief, rank those ideas by risk, starting with the lowest risk ways. List only ways that are within a reasonable risk. *Do not list any high-risk ways to collect evidence.*

Belief: _____

Alternative interpretation: _____

Least Feared Actions/Observations

_____

_____

_____

_____

_____

_____

_____

_____

_____

_____

Most Feared Actions/Observations

She didn't carry out her plan right away. She thought about it for awhile and found some further ways to reduce the risk. For example, it was helpful to plan the sort of situation that might be best for mentioning a piece of information. She also had to consider how to keep an open mind as her friend reacted. What sort of reaction meant acceptance to Ellen? Was it the way her friend expressed acceptance? Ellen decided she needed check out how her friend expressed acceptance before doing anything risky that relied on getting an accepting response. She brainstormed questions she might ask her friend and decided to have a general conversation about how each of them communicated acceptance. When she did this, she learned a lot about her friend and about how her friend read her. Knowing more about how to read her friend's response also helped her lower the risk for revealing information about her past. When she felt comfortable, she slowly, at her own pace, carried out her plan of revealing information about her past. She kept track of the accumulating evidence by recording it on Exercises 8.10 and 8.11 (see pages 309 and 310). Gradually, the weight of the evidence accumulated that the friend was indeed accepting Ellen's revelations.

SUMMARIZING YOUR WORK ON INTIMACY

Consider now what you need for yourself. You can put this workbook aside for now, or you can continue to work on it as you choose. Feel free to identify other beliefs about intimacy, evaluate them, and test how accurate they may be. When you are you ready to stop your work on intimacy for the time being, fill out Exercise 8.12 as a summary of your work. You can return to issues of intimacy at any time. Reviewing this summary when you come back will give you a sense of where you can restart your work.

We also suggest that you revisit earlier parts of this workbook. When you review the text and exercises on the other needs, you may well be able to see connections among them that you did not see the first time. New thoughts may come to mind that prove helpful to you. Over time, you can continue to build on your work.

As you leave your work on intimacy, even if briefly, remember that intimacy usually takes time to grow. For intimacy to grow, you need to risk

EXERCISE 8.10   What Evidence Do I Have about the Existing Belief?

What evidence do you already have about the accuracy of your existing belief? What facts, words, or actions support the belief? What facts, words, or actions indicate the belief is inaccurate? Write those down below.

Belief: _____

What facts or evidence support this belief as accurate?

1. _____
2. _____
3. _____

What facts or evidence indicate this belief is not accurate?

1. _____
2. _____
3. _____

How sure are you that this belief is accurate? Mark how sure on the following scale. Use the second evaluation scale later to check on changes in your beliefs in light of new evidence.

Date: _____

Accurate   Inaccurate

_____

100%   50%   0%

Date: _____

Accurate   Inaccurate

_____

100%   50%   0%

✿ EXERCISE 8.11   What Evidence Do I Have about the Alternative Meaning?

What evidence do you already have about the accuracy of the alternative meaning? What facts, words, or actions support the alternative meaning? What facts, words, or actions indicate the alternative meaning is inaccurate? Write those down below.

Alternative meaning: _____

What facts or evidence support this interpretation as accurate?

1. _____
2. _____
3. _____

What facts or evidence indicate this interpretation is not accurate?

1. _____
2. _____
3. _____

How sure are you that this interpretation is accurate? Mark how sure on the following scale. Use the second evaluation scale later to check on changes in your beliefs in light of new evidence.

Date: _____

Accurate   Inaccurate

_____

100%   50%   0%

Date: _____

Accurate   Inaccurate

_____

100%   50%   0%

EXERCISE 8.12 Summarizing Your Work on Intimacy

I have identified the following beliefs about intimacy:

I can think of the following alternative meanings:

I have already carried out the following steps (mark with X); or I would like in the future to carry out the following steps (mark with *):

_____ Make a list of what evidence might confirm and/or contradict the existing belief.

_____ Organize the list of evidence from least feared/least risky to collect to most feared/most risky to collect.

_____ Carry out the least feared/least risky way to collect evidence.

_____ Keep a record of the evidence collected—both pro and con.

List here any evidence collected—what did you see or do, and how did it turn out? Continue adding to this list over time, as you become aware of additional evidence.

letting yourself be known. Also, you have to recognize acceptance from others when they offer it. True intimacy requires that you already have some measure of safety, trust, control, and self-esteem. Once some small measure of intimacy is achieved, it helps strengthen your ability to get these other needs met.

HEALING FOR THE LONG TERM

This workbook is coming to an end, but it is not the end of your healing journey. The work described in this book is intended to be done over the long term. Our needs for safety, trust, self-esteem, power, and intimacy are life-long and keep changing as we change and grow.

COPING WITH STRESS

Day-to-day life after trauma can be difficult, but life can get easier, especially when you remember and use the 10 effective ways of coping with stress first described in Chapter 2. We have built these 10 strategies into the individual chapters. We want to list them again for you now to remind you of some of the ways they can be used.

Ten Effective Ways to Cope with Stress
1. Be flexible, try new things, experiment.
2. Learn all you can about what is going to happen.
3. Plan ahead.
4. Avoid impulsive changes.
5. Try not to change too many things at once.
6. Pay attention to your reactions and feelings.
7. Talk to others who have survived similar experiences.
8. Seek support from people who can listen.
9. Allow yourself to grieve losses.
10. Take your time.

Be Flexible, Think Flexibly

Leftover fear from trauma can restrict your creativity and narrow your range of options. From where you stand, you may only be able to see one course of action. But if you shift your position, your view changes. Thinking flexibly means being able to see things from new or different perspectives rather than from the same old one. When you do this, new thoughts and choices become visible that were hard to see before. Being able to talk with others can be a big help in thinking more flexibly.

> ❁ *Diane blamed herself for not being able to save her sister from drowning when they were both children. For years she was tortured with questions about why she had lived and her sister had not. Eventually one of Diane's friends asked her what it was like for her to go through the boating accident. What was it like for her to be caught in the strong waves and not know if she would survive? This question made Diane consider her experience from the outside, from her friend's and her own adult perspective. For the first time Diane realized how dangerous and difficult a situation she had been in, and yet she was only a child. She felt enormous empathy for the child she had been. She realized that it was a terrifying experience for anyone to have gone through. She continued to have painful feelings when she thought of the accident. But she no longer blamed herself so harshly for what happened.*

Learn All You Can about What Is Going to Happen

Fear and stress make it more difficult to think flexibly, but gathering as much information as you can—in advance—can help you stay flexible and see your full range of choices. You may fear something will happen, but how do the facts of the current situation match your emotions? What can you learn about the situation? The more you know in advance, the more choices you can have, and the more you can feel in control.

> ❁ *Jean always felt afraid and anxious going to the gynecologist. The exams evoked strong images and feelings that reminded her of being sexually abused by a neighbor as a child. It became even more difficult when she had to schedule more frequent and uncomfortable procedures to treat her difficulty in getting pregnant. Although it was never easy, she found it very*

helpful to learn as much as she could about each procedure before it happened. She did this by reading, talking to her doctor, and attending an infertility group.

Plan Ahead

When you have gathered information about something that might happen, you can begin to consider, in advance, what you can do to prepare. Perhaps there are ways to make it easier for you. When you plan ahead, you plan when you can still think clearly and flexibly, before the highest level of stress. What will you need at those moments of peak stress? What might help you? How can you have these people or things handy? You can create a plan of action to make things easier for you and as safe as possible.

Avoid Impulsive Changes

Impulsive change can put you at risk. Respect your needs for safety. Try to think things through before you act. This gives you a better sense of control and power in the situation and can help you keep your risk low.

Try Not to Change Too Many Things at Once

You have the power to change many things about yourself, your behavior, and your reactions to others. Using this power most effectively means knowing its limitations. Changes, even good ones, create stress. The more changes, the more stress, and therefore, the harder it is to stay flexible. Changing too many things at once can overload you and make everything harder. You can end up feeling out of control. You can feel more in control by not changing too many things at once.

Pay Attention to Your Feelings and Reactions

You need to value and respect yourself enough to listen to how you feel. Paying attention to yourself gives you basic, crucial information. It is part of how you learn what is happening inside you. It is how you know whether or not you are changing too much, going too fast, or taking too many risks. Paying attention to yourself can give you the information and evidence that you need to plan ahead for next time.

Talk to Others Who Have Survived Similar Changes or Experiences

Trauma can result in powerful, uncomfortable feelings of being crazy, separate, and different from others. It is even more powerful in a comforting way to realize you are not alone. After not knowing whom to talk to or how to put your experiences into words, it can be tremendously healing to learn there are others who understand and can share what you have been through. Talking to others who have had similar experiences also helps you get back in touch with yourself, and accept yourself.

❀ *At the age of 65, Cecilia was diagnosed with a severe form of cancer. She and her family went through the painful early stages of shock, disbelief, and terror. Over the early weeks following her diagnosis, Cecilia felt many confusing and painful things. She also started to feel that those closest to her could not really understand what it was like for her. In addition, she started feeling protective of them and stopped sharing the most difficult of her fears and other emotional experiences. Soon she learned of a support network for cancer patients and started attending a support group. She found it was easier to speak openly with other people going through similar experiences. She was immediately relieved just to know she was not alone in her feelings about her illness or about her relationships.*

Seek Support from People Who Can Listen, Offer Feedback, or Help in Other Ways

Everyone needs help sometime for something. When you can begin to count on others for help, it takes a great load off your shoulders. Finding people you can trust for even small, low-risk, practical things is a start. Finding people who will listen and accept you for who you are is one of the greatest supports of all.

Allow Yourself to Grieve Losses

Trauma and change bring loss. Although uncomfortable and at times, even unbearable, the pain of loss can be one way to acknowledge and respect what you value. Pain confirms that what was lost was important to you and mattered. Respecting your feelings means that you have value, you matter, and continue to matter, even through loss.

Take Your Time

Healing from trauma can mean rebuilding your life. You need time to do this safely and solidly. Take the time. If you listen to your feelings and reactions, and respect what they tell you, you will move as fast as you can. Remember that you cannot control everything. If you try to go faster than your own limits allow, it will slow you down in the end.

The above ways of coping work for any stress, not just trauma. They are valuable tools for the rest of your life. We recognize that nothing erases trauma's tragedy and pain, but the experience as a whole can also include the silver linings of positive change and personal growth.

GROWING STRONGER

I survived what no-one could survive. That is the strength I discovered in myself. . . . Now I know I can do anything, and I know I want to choose very much more carefully what I will do. Each moment is precious. My life is precious. . . . Each person . . . is precious. I knew that before, but I wanted security most. I discovered I am strong enough to face the reality that there is no security, and to jump over the edge and live fully.
—Brenda R. Shaw

Recognizing Your Strengths

The very fact that you survived, whatever your physical and emotional condition, reflects your strength. Following a traumatic experience, some people are stunned to consider what they have lived through. "How did I do it?" "I never imagined I could handle such as thing." "I can't believe I survived that." These are common thoughts that survivors have. No matter how bad things were or how difficult things continue to be, you have been able to go on living. After a trauma, you may recognize your strength and resilience in ways that were never apparent before. You may find that you are stronger than you thought you were. You may find that you have gained new knowledge, insight, or wisdom from your experience.

> ❀ *Rona was 37 when her husband, John, was killed in a sudden, tragic accident. She was left alone to raise their two children. John had been the financial provider and primary decision maker in the family. She had always seen him as stronger than she was. She had lacked the confidence to make major decisions so looked to him to take the lead. After John's death, Rona went through a period of mourning and self-exploration. Gradually, she began to recognize that she had ideas, opinions, and feelings of her own. Over time, she became more confident and started to enjoy making decisions and planning the family's activities. She never stopped missing her husband or grieving his loss, but she felt excited by the unexpected changes in herself.*

Rona suffered a great loss and much pain. As she healed she realized that this terrible situation had also led her to gain insight and new skills. She realized that she had strength that she had not appreciated before.

> ❀ *Elaine, a survivor of childhood abuse, did not learn about her strengths until she was an adult, long after the abuse ended. As a child she had suffered brutal attacks by her father, which left her feeling that everything about her was bad and contaminated. When she was able to examine the effect of the abuse in a safe and supportive relationship, Elaine began to recognize that understanding her own pain led to a deepened compassion for others. Out of her suffering grew a gift for helping others. She had possessed this strength before but had not recognized it as the strength it really was.*

Has your recovery from trauma led you to see strengths in yourself you did not see before? What strengths do you recognize in yourself as a result of your experience?

Bringing Your Life Into Focus

A traumatic event can suddenly make crystal clear what is and is not important to you. Your priorities in life can shift. The time, thought, and energy you commit to certain activities and relationships can change.

❧ *Andy was in an extremely serious automobile accident. The emergency crews at the accident scene had to cut Andy and his friend out of the car, amazed that they had survived. After several months of physical recovery, Andy recognized a shift in his attitudes. He stopped answering phone calls from casual friends with whom he used to drink beer but in whom he had no real interest. Instead, he focused on a few meaningful friendships with people who could talk about feelings and experiences. He also kept in contact with the hospital unit where he had spent part of his recovery. He sometimes spoke with other accident victims who needed support.*

Have you noticed any shift in your priorities since your trauma? If so, how?

Achieving Emotional Freedom

Being deluged with feelings may initially feel unwelcome, scary, dangerous, or otherwise overwhelming. Over time, however, you can learn to know and express your feelings in a positive way. Knowing and expressing your feelings helps you understand yourself, take better care of yourself, provides you with relief and allows more closeness in your relationships.

❧ *When Dana was a teenager, her father had stabbed and injured her boyfriend, though not fatally. Dana didn't want to lose her closeness with her father, but trying to hold onto it kept her from fully sorting out the confusion of rage and grief that she felt. It wasn't until Dana was an adult that she began to speak about what happened and how she felt. When she began speaking openly about the stabbing, she was surprised to find it became easier to speak more openly about other things as well. Her closest relationships became closer than they had been. She felt less anxious and more confident in other areas of her life.*

Do you feel more able to know and express your feelings since starting this workbook? Has that been positive in any way?

TOWARD A GREATER MEANING

Throughout this workbook, we have talked about the possible meanings of specific facts, events, and needs. But many human beings also seek and need a larger sense of meaning in their lives. Why do things happen? Do events occur randomly or do they have a purpose? Does human life have an overarching meaning? If so, what is it? Why are we here?

Different people give different names to their sense of greater meaning and it can take different forms. Sometimes it is called a *worldview* or *life philosophy*. This can include values and moral principles as well as beliefs about why things happen. Sometimes this sense takes the form of traditional religion or a less formal spirituality. By *spirituality*, we mean the belief that there is a dimension of experience greater than you, and beyond you, which also exists within you. This could include awareness of the nonmaterial, existential aspects of experience, your sense of life's meaning, or a striving toward personal growth. Your sense of life's larger meaning can be disrupted by trauma. Restoring or rebuilding this meaning can be as important a part of healing as regaining any of the other needs discussed in this book.

❀ *Carlos was on a routine flight from his home in Miami to his parents' home in South America. His plane came in for a landing, but when it was about 200 feet above water, it lost engine power and fell. Carlos was not a good swimmer and thought he was about to die. The plane quickly submerged about 20 feet. Carlos lost consciousness on impact and then came to under the water. He noticed that the emergency exits were open and some people were swimming out of the plane. Everyone seated around him was dead. Carlos undid his seat belt but began to lose consciousness again from lack of air. Suddenly a bubble of white light surrounded him. The bubble carried him to the plane's exit and almost to the water's surface before it disappeared. He was met at the surface by emergency personnel who had responded quickly. Carlos believes that he was rescued from certain death by a spiritual being or power. He sees this new chance for life as a way to work for others. He has become an advocate of airline safety and started taking courses in psychology. He has some nightmares, but is able to fly regularly. He always asks for an exit row seat, and still has some anxiety during landings but generally feels at peace when he thinks of the accident.*

If you have a strong sense of spirituality, you may have an enduring sense of hope, a deep awareness of the nonmaterial aspects of life, and a sense of connection with something or someone beyond yourself. You may feel support from these beliefs as they help you move through painful feelings. Your spirituality may serve as a means to soothe you and give you a sense of connection.

❦ *Kayla's source of strength through abuse and recovery was her connection with nature. She grew up with an unpredictable and very violent mother. If Kayla showed any reaction after being beaten, such as crying, her mother usually became angrier, yelling and hitting her more. Kayla recalls a time when she locked herself in her room after one of these incidents and stared out the window. It was raining. She felt the sky was crying with her, grieving for her pain. Her connection with nature was the only relationship she could count on during those years and it helped sustain her. It gave her a sense of spiritual connection with the world that meant she was not totally alone with her pain.*

You may want to consider your own beliefs about life's larger meaning. Do you believe there is a level of experience that exists beyond the sensory, physical, or mental?

Has your spiritual life helped you cope with or heal from trauma?

Has your spiritual life changed as a result of your traumatic experiences? If so, in what ways?

If your views have shifted over time, how do you understand the change?

What role do you hope spirituality might have in your future?

Do you have a sense of hope for the future?

From where does that hope come?

Healing from a trauma can have unpredictable and far-reaching effects, including benefits. They may not make you glad for the traumatic experience, but they may leave you with unexpected gifts. The following is a list of possible gifts. Please add your own experiences to the list.

Gifts That Can Come as You Recover from Trauma
- New awareness of your inner strength
- Different set of priorities
- Heightened appreciation for daily life
- Respect for others who have survived trauma
- Sense of awe at nature and the cycles of life
- Deepened emotional life

- Deepened spiritual life
- A philosophy of life that explains tragedy and makes sense of the unexpected
- Comfort with or acceptance of what once was too frightening to contemplate
- Understanding of life's complexities
- Confidence that you can survive anything

- _____
- _____
- _____

It is possible that you cannot yet imagine recovering from trauma or believe there can be any unexpected gifts. What you notice about yourself will change over time. In the initial period following trauma, grief and other difficult emotions need to be addressed. After some time, other aspects of your experience, including what has been gained, may emerge. Take the time that you need for yourself and you can get to this point.

CONCLUSION

As you continue your healing journey, stay flexible, and remember there are no givens or absolutes in our world. The circumstances of your life will change and keep changing. You will be faced with new situations and demands, but you can return at any time to the strategies and resources that you have found most supportive, helpful and nurturing whether they are from this book or elsewhere.

My Song
I have walked the road
That many have never walked
I have seen things
That you can't imagine
I have heard the cries of angels
And never knew they were my own

My steps were labored
Wondering why I was not among the favored
Dreading each day
Trying to hold the monsters at bay

But through it all I kept hearing that song
That sweet melody playing in my brain
It was a song of hope
Its words spoke of courage
Its sweetness spoke of life
And when I awake each day
I am filled with this song
My song
The song of hope

by Patricia Nelson and Janille Johnson
Reprinted by permission of *Coping* magazine

RECOMMENDED READINGS

SELF-CARE

Davis, M., E. R. Eshelman, and M. McKay. *The Relaxation and Stress Reduction Workbook*. Oakland, CA: New Harbinger, 1995.

Gershon, D., and G. Strauss. *Empowerment: The Art of Creating Your Life as You Want It*. New York: Dell, 1989.

Greenberger, Dennis, and Christine Padesky. *Mind Over Mood: Change How You Feel by Changing the Way You Think*. New York: Guilford Press, 1995.

Louden, Jennifer. *The Woman's Comfort Book: A Self-Nurturing Guide for Restoring Balance in Your Life*. San Francisco: Harper San Francisco, 1992.

Miller, Dusty. *Women Who Hurt Themselves: A Book of Hope and Understanding*. New York: Basic Books, 1994.

Pines, A. *Burnout: Handbook of Stress*. New York: The Free Press, 1993.

Siegel, R. S. *Six Seconds to True Calm*. Santa Monica, CA: Little Sun Books, 1995.

Zi, Nancy. *The Art of Breathing: Exercises for Improving Your Performance and Well-Being*. New York: Bantam, 1986.

Zuercher-White, E. *An End to Panic: Breakthrough Techniques for Overcoming Panic Disorder*. Oakland, CA: New Harbinger Publications, 1995.

GENERAL TRAUMA

Flannery, Raymond B. *Post-Traumatic Stress Disorder: The Victim's Guide to Healing and Recovery*. Holyoke, MA: Crossroad, 1992.

Herman, Judith Lewis. *Trauma and Recovery*. New York: Basic Books, 1992.

Matsakis, Aphrodite. *I Can't Get over It: A Handbook for Trauma Survivors*. Oakland, CA: New Harbinger, 1992.

McCann, Lisa, and Laurie Ann Pearlman, *Psychological Trauma and the Adult Survivor.* New York: Brunner/Mazel, 1990.

Miller, D. *Women Who Hurt Themselves: A Book of Hope and Understanding.* New York: Basic Books, 1994.

LOSS AND GRIEF

Fitzgerald, Helen. *The Mourning Handbook: A Complete Guide for the Bereaved.* Upper Saddle River, NJ: Simon & Schuster, 1994.

James, John and Frank Cherry. *The Grief Recovery Handbook.* New York: HarperCollins, 1989.

Marcus, Eric. *Why Suicide?* New York: HarperCollins, 1996.

Quinnett, Paul G. *Suicide: The Forever Decision.* Holyoke, MA: Crossroad, 1987.

Rosof, Barbara D. *The Worst Loss.* New York: Henry Holt, 1994.

Tatelbaum, Judy. *The Courage to Grieve.* New York: HarperCollins, 1984.

Weenolsen, Patricia. *The Art of Dying.* New York: St. Martins, 1996.

HELPING CHILDREN COPE WITH LOSS AND GRIEF

Fitzgerald, Helen. *The Grieving Child.* Old Tappan, NJ: Fireside, 1992.

Grollman, Earl A. *Straight Talk about Death for Teenagers: How to Cope with Losing Someone You Love.* Boston: Beacon, 1993.

Mellonie, Bryan, and Robert Ingpen. *Lifetimes: The Beautiful Way to Explain Death to Children.* New York: Bantam Doubleday Dell, 1987.

ABUSE

Ackerman, Robert J., and Susan E. Pickering. *Before It's Too Late.* Deerfield Beach, FL: Health Communications, 1995.

Bean, Barbara, and Shari Bennett. *The Me Nobody Knows: A Guide for Teen Survivors.* Columbus, OH: Lexington, 1993.

Dutton, Donald G. *The Batterer: A Psychological Profile.* New York : Basic Books, 1995.

Gil, Eliana. *Outgrowing the Pain Together: A Book for Spouses and Partners of Adults Abused as Children.* New York: Dell, 1992.

Hunter, Mic. *Abused Boys.* New York: Ballantine, 1990.

Ledray, Linda E. *Recovering from Rape.* New York: Henry Holt, 1986.

Lew, Mike. *Victims No Longer: Men Recovering from Incest and Other Sexual Child Abuse.* New York: HarperCollins, 1990.

Middleton-Moz, Jane. *Children of Trauma: Rediscovering Your Discarded Self.* Deerfield, FL: Health Communications, 1989.

Napier, Nancy J. *Getting through the Day: Strategies for Adults Hurt as Children.* New York: W.W. Norton, 1993.

Sanford, Linda T. *Strong at the Broken Places: Overcoming the Trauma of Childhood Abuse.* New York: Random House, 1990.

SAFETY

Williams, M. B. "Establishing Safety in Survivors of Severe Sexual Abuse in Posttraumatic Stress Therapy." *Treating Abuse Today* 3(1): 4–11, 1993.

Williams, M. B. "Establishing Safety in Survivors of Severe Sexual Abuse in Posttraumatic Stress Therapy, Part II." *Treating Abuse Today* 3(2): 13–16, 1993.

Williams, M. B. "Establishing Safety in Survivors of Severe Sexual Abuse in Posttraumatic Stress Therapy, Part III." *Treating Abuse Today* 3(3): 13–14, 1993.

Williams, M. B. "Helping Survivors Retrieve Memories and Avoid Self-Destructive Behavior." *Moving Forward* 2(1): 8–9, 11, Nov./Dec. 1992.

Williams, M. B. "Taking the Sense of Safety Beyond the Therapy Setting." *Moving Forward* 2(2): 6–7, Jan./Feb. 1993.

TRUST

Jampolsky, Lee. *The Art of Trust.* Berkeley, CA: Celestial Arts, 1994.

Williams, M. B. "Post-Traumatic Therapy: Fostering Trust and Empowering Survivors." *Moving Forward* 1(4): 8–9, Sept./Oct. 1992.

EMPOWERMENT

Alberti, R. E., and M. L. Emmons. *Your Perfect Right: A Guide to Assertive Living.* 5th ed. San Luis Obispo, CA: Impact Publishers, 1986.

Janeway, Elizabeth. *The Powers of the Weak.* New York: Knopf, 1980.

SELF-ESTEEM

Branden, Nathaniel. *The Power of Self-Esteem.* Deerfield Beach, FL: Health Communications, 1992.

Branden, Nathaniel. *The Six Pillars of Self-Esteem.* New York: Bantam Doubleday Dell, 1995.

McKay, Matthew, and Patrick Fanning. *Respecting Your Emotional Life.* New York: Fine Communications, 1994.

INTIMACY

Carter, Steven, and Julia Sokol. *He's Scared, She's Scared.* New York: Dell, 1995.

Dixon, Monica. *Love the Body You Were Born With.* New York: Berkley, 1996.

Katherine, Anne. *Boundaries: Where You End and I Begin.*
Old Tappan, NJ: Fireside, 1993.

Lerner, Harriet. *The Dance of Intimacy, A Woman's Guide to Courageous Acts of Change in Key Relationships.* San Francisco: Harper, 1989.

Louden, Jennifer. *The Couples Comfort Book.* San Farancisco, CA: Harper, 1994.

Prochelo, Barbara. *Draw from Within: A Workbook for Self-Expression and Self-Discovery.* Scottsdale, AZ: SunDance Creations, 1990.

Whitfield, Charles L. *Boundaries and Relationships.* Deerfield Beach FL: Health Communications, 1993.

SPIRITUALITY

The Foundation for Inner Peace, *A Course in Miracles.* New York: Viking Penguin, 1996.

Moore, Thomas. *Care of the Soul.* San Francisco: Harper Perennial, 1994.

Moore, Thomas. *The Reenchantment of Everyday Life.* New York: HarperCollins, 1996.

Muller, Wayne. *How, Then, Shall We Live?* New York: Bantam, 1996.

Wakefield, Dan. *Expect a Miracle.* New York: Walker, 1995.

Walsch, N. D. *Conversations with God: An Uncommon Dialogue.* New York: Penguin Putnam, 1996.

PARENTING

While this was not a focus in our workbook, parenting can be profoundly affected by traumatic experiences. Individuals who grow up in a traumatic context, such as an abusive or very neglectful family, may not learn certain tools to parent the way they would like. It's common to parent the way you were parented; there are times that you may want to do something differently but do not know what or how. Here are some helpful resources for all parents. Some address communication and others help provide an understanding of what to expect at various ages.

Faber, Adele, and Elaine Mazlish. *How to Talk So Kids Will Listen and Listen So Kids Will Talk.* New York: Avon, 1980.

Joslin, Karen Renshaw. *Positive Parenting from A to Z.* New York: Fawcett, 1994.

Vannoy, Steven W. *The 10 Greatest Gifts I Give My Children: Parenting from the Heart.* Old Tappan, NJ: Fireside, 1994.

Wolf, Anthony E. *Get Out of My Life, but First Could You Drive Me and Cheryl to the Mall? A Parent's Guide to the New Teenager.* New York: Noonday Press, 1991.

For parents who are concerned that they may be mistreating or abusing their child or might be at risk for hurting their child, confidential information and help is available through calling 1-800-CHILDREN; this national number will route you to a local 1-800 number. The phones are generally staffed from 9:00 AM–5:00 PM, weekdays, but this may vary from one city to another. After hours, you may contact your local Department for Children and Families.

About Psychotherapy

Not everyone needs psychotherapy following a trauma, but it can often be helpful. Entering psychotherapy does *not* mean that the person who seeks help must be crazy or sick. Most people in psychotherapy are struggling with common life challenges and are seeking help for a variety of problems they may not be able to solve on their own. Therapy can be helpful for those who want to sort out difficult experiences in the present or past such as traumatic experiences. It can help people to understand and manage confusing or painful feelings such as sadness, anxiety, anger, or low self-esteem.

Psychotherapy is not about getting advice. A therapist will listen to your problems and help you draw your own conclusions about how to solve them. He or she does not have all the answers but will have some useful questions or thoughts. She or he will offer observations about how thoughts and feelings connect to each other as well as to present and past experiences. Issues of safety, trust, control, esteem, and intimacy will usually arise. Although psychotherapy often becomes an emotionally intimate relationship in which you can feel listened to and accepted for being yourself, physical intimacy is off-limits. It is unethical for a therapist to become physically intimate with any client.

Psychotherapy can be difficult work. Sometimes people go through strong and painful feelings on their way to becoming healthier. Clients may feel worse before feeling better. But psychotherapy does work to make most clients feel better.

SUGGESTIONS FOR FINDING A THERAPIST FOR TRAUMA

Most states license psychotherapists and this licensing requires some basic level of training. However, this training may not include work with trauma survivors. If you are considering psychotherapy for a specific problem, it is important to find a therapist with good professional qualifications plus experience in that problem area. This is especially true for help in recovering from a traumatic experience. There are three important things to look for in finding a psychotherapist for help with any traumatic experience.

1. The therapist needs to be qualified to do psychotherapy.
2. The therapist needs to have specialized training and experience in working with trauma survivors.
3. You need to feel there is a good fit between your personality and that of the therapist.

Basic Psychotherapist Qualifications

Psychotherapy is practiced by a range of mental health professionals. Psychotherapists may have a professional degree in social work (MA, MSW), psychology (PhD, PsyD), psychiatry (MD), counseling (EdD), or nursing (MSN). Any therapist who treats trauma survivors should have some specific training in treating trauma. Not all therapists have such training.

Feeling a Good Fit with the Therapist

Psychotherapy works best when there is a good fit between your personality and that of the therapist. A therapist may be extremely well qualified and work well with many people but his or her personality could rub yours the wrong way. It is no one's fault when this happens, but when it does that person is not the best therapist for you; look for someone else. It is good to get at least two names of possible therapists when asking for referrals. You can check out both of them to see which one fits you best. Briefly interview both on the telephone. Ask them about their professional training and their specialized training and experience with trauma. A telephone conversation can give you some information about the kind of person each therapist is. The best way, however, is to make an appointment to meet with each one before deciding with whom to work. Consider the following kinds of questions: Is she or he a good listener? Does the therapist seem to understand what I am talking about and how I am feeling? Does the therapist seem to know what she or he is doing? If your answer to all these questions is "yes" then that person is probably a good therapist for you.

Finding a Psychotherapist Trained for Trauma Recovery

Finding a therapist with experience and training in trauma is important. However, there is no single recommended route and no single degree or credential that a good trauma therapist always has. You can probably locate a trained trauma therapist in your area by contacting the following organizations and asking for names in your geographical area.

Association of Traumatic Stress Specialists (ATSS)
> 7338 Broad River Road
> Irmo, SC 29063
> 803-781-0017 Fax: 803-781-3899

> ATSS is an international, nonprofit membership organization founded in 1989 to provide certification and professional education to those actively involved in trauma response, treatment, management, and crisis organization. The association maintains an international list of skilled crisis responders, trainees, therapists, debriefers, and others. The initials CTS and CTR indicate such certification.

ISSD
> International Society for the Study of Dissociation
> 60 Revere Drive, Suite 500
> Northbrook, IL 60062
> 847-480-0899 Fax: 847-480-9282

Sidran Foundation—Publishing Company and Catalog of PTSD related
> books
> Esther Giller, Director
> 2328 W. Joppa Road, Suite 15
> Lutherville, MD 21093
> 410-825-8888

American Psychological Association
> 750 First Street, NE

Washington, DC 20002-4242
202-336-5500

This is the national professional organization for psychologists. Each state also has its own association that can refer you to psychotherapists in your geographic area. Be sure to ask for a therapist who has experience treating trauma survivors. If your state psychological association is not in your phone book, the national association can give it to you.

National Association of Social Workers
750 First Street NE, Suite 700
Washington, DC 20002-4241
1-800-742-4089

The Traumatology Institute
Bruce Manciagli
CPD/FSU
Tallahassee, FL 32306-1640
805-644-1966 Fax: 850-644-2589

Other Resources

International Society for Traumatic Stress Studies
60 Revere Drive, Suite 500
Northbrook, IL 60062
847-480-9028

This is an organization for professionals from multiple disciplines interested in sharing advances in trauma research, theory, treatment strategies, and public policy. The organization has developed a resource pamphlet that can be sent out on request.

"Trauma Information Pages" on the World Wide Web
http://www.trauma-pages.com/

Dr. David Baldwin is a psychologist who maintains this Web site. The Web site includes information on treatments for trauma as well as links to many other trauma-related Web sites.

PTSDisorders Internet Forum
    Charles Figley
    traumatic-stress@LISTP.APA.ORG

This Internet forum is for professionals and survivors. Subscribers discuss a variety of trauma-related information upon request.

Trauma Counseling Certificate Program
    University of Alabama
    College of Continuing Studies
    Box 870388
    Tuscaloosa, AL 35487-0388
    205-348-6225

10 days of instruction divided into four blocks; earns credits for CTS (Certified Trauma Specialist) from ATSS. Contact person: Geri Stone.

APPENDIX C

Comments for Mental Health Professionals on How to Use This Workbook

This workbook is intended for use by trauma survivors, on their own, outside a therapy context. However, it might also be valuable when used properly within therapy. If you or your client are interested in using the workbook in conjunction with psychotherapy, we offer a few guidelines, suggestions, and cautions for making the safest and most effective use of this material.

THE WORKBOOK'S THERAPEUTIC USES AND LIMITATIONS

This book's focus is on the survivor's posttrauma present. Its purpose is to help survivors cope with the disorienting symptoms typical in the aftermath of a trauma. This book is *not* a guide to working through the trauma itself. We repeatedly advise readers against evoking trauma memories or using those memories for the exercises in this book. While aspects of the text may unavoidably trigger flashbacks or memories of the trauma, we advise readers to turn immediately to calming and self-comforting activities when this happens.

> **Caution**
>
> **If you have no specialized training in trauma, do not attempt to evoke or examine traumatic memories.** Please observe the same cautions we have given to survivors. Help keep the client focused on the present. Use this book as a way to help survivors recover and strengthen basic coping strategies in their present daily lives. This is the first priority for any trauma survivor. Survivors risk retraumatization and harm from examination of trauma memories if done improperly, without appropriate guidance from a specially trained professional.

THEORY AND RESEARCH ON WHICH THIS WORKBOOK IS BASED

The premise of this workbook is that trauma disrupts cognitive schemas, or beliefs, about self and others in five areas of psychological need: safety, trust, control, esteem, and intimacy. This workbook invites survivors to rebuild their coping resources in the short term through self-care and self-comforting, and then to rebuild them in the longer term through rethinking the posttrauma meaning of these needs.

The basic concept that trauma disrupts beliefs in five need areas is based on constructivist self-development theory (McCann & Pearlman, 1990; Pearlman and Saakvitne, 1995). This theory draws upon and integrates self-psychology, object relations, interpersonal, and social cognition theories. The information on coping and self-care is drawn from wide range of coping and stress research and literature such as Aldwin and Revenson, 1987; Carver et al; 1989; Dunkel-Schetter et al; 1992; Lazarus and Folkman, 1984; Lazarus, 1993; Resick and Schnicke, 1993; Dattilio and Freeman, 1994; Padesky and Greenberger, 1995; Slaby, 1988.

HOW TO PROCEED IN THE WORKBOOK

Trauma survivors need to begin at the beginning of the workbook. The first three chapters of the workbook are designed to give survivors basic skills and techniques for self-comforting and coping with symptoms. Clients need to have these coping resources for emotional safety before moving past

Chapter 3. Clients should have several techniques that work for them before moving further. Once the client has basic coping techniques in place, the need chapters (Chapters 4 through 8) can be started.

The most important need for any survivor is safety. The need for safety, Chapter 4, should be the first need assessed and addressed. This chapter includes discussion and additional techniques for emotional safety as well as physical safety. It is important for clients to have effective strategies for maintaining their emotional safety before moving beyond this chapter. The subsequent chapters build on each other, but they need not be addressed in sequence. If the main issue is clearly self-esteem, for example, then you and the survivor together may decide to move directly to that chapter after the safety chapter.

ASSESSMENT SUGGESTIONS

For each of the five basic needs covered, this book provides a number of exercises for informal self-assessment of the survivor' beliefs. These exercises should give you and your client a sense of which needs have been disrupted by the trauma, which are problematic and which are not. For a more statistically meaningful, formal assessment, we recommend Traumatic Stress Institute's Belief Scale. It is available through Western Psychological Services, 12031 Wilshire Boulevard, Los Angeles, CA 90025-1251.

TIMING AND PACING IN USING THE WORKBOOK

The key to using the workbook effectively is to help the client take her or his time and not hurry. Some clients may want to tackle a chapter of the workbook for each session. This can be overwhelming and counterproductive. Help clients slow down and encourage them to attend to their feelings and reactions as a guide for how fast to move. Learning to attend to feelings is a crucial lesson in this workbook.

Talk with clients about their answers to the exercises and questions. What do the answers mean? Can the client begin to identify some beliefs and recognize whether those beliefs are problematic? It can be helpful for clients to complete some of the exercises during the therapy session. Discussing responses with clients can help open them to new views of the issues at hand. When doing the exercises, take care to steer them toward current issues and problems and away from traumatic events or memories.

Taking time to notice and discuss emotions that arise when reflecting on certain beliefs or experiences is also critical to the healing process. Therapy can provide a uniquely safe place to do this work.

Help the client know when to take a break from the workbook. The text may trigger memories, affects, or insights. Thus it is important to help a client cope with traumatic stress reactions and regain a sense of stability before moving ahead. The client may need brief or extended time periods to process these materials before moving on further in the workbook.

If your client is making use of this workbook independently, be sure to review work that the client has done at home. Ask questions about intrusive thoughts, emotions, and/or flashbacks that the client may have while working at home. Help the client manage and process these when they occur. If you are using workbook content within therapy sessions be sure to allow time at the end of sessions to process or step back from the intense emotions stirred up during the session. Examples of relaxation exercises are included in this book at the ends of Chapters 1, 2, and 3. You may wish to make tapes of one or more of them for your client to take home. A tape of a relaxation exercise in your voice can be very reassuring. Other strategies for ending sessions include leaving time at the end to check in with the client about how he or she is feeling and what he or she might need to do for self-care following the session.

BE AWARE OF YOUR OWN BELIEFS

If you use this workbook with clients, it is important to become aware of your own beliefs about safety, trust, control, self-esteem, and intimacy. Your beliefs influence how you act in sessions and how you respond to your client's beliefs around these issues.

A few issues for therapists concerning personal needs include the following: Do you feel vulnerable to harm? How do you protect yourself as you do this work? Is your office a safe place for you? Do you believe you are a trustworthy person? Do you conduct your practice in ways that help trust develop by operating in a predictable manner with established boundaries? Do you respect and not abuse the power of your position as a therapist?

KNOW WHEN REFERRAL IS APPROPRIATE

If therapy with a particular client feels problematic and moves beyond your training and expertise, you should seek supervision or consultation. If the therapy continues to feel stuck or unproductive, consider facilitating a referral to a qualified trauma therapist. This is best done in a planned and supportive way that blames neither the client nor therapist.

We hope you and your clients will find this workbook helpful. We welcome feedback from both you and your clients including any suggestions you might have for future editions of this workbook. Send comments to Dena Rosenbloom, in care of the Guilford Press, 72 Spring Street, New York, New York 10012, or by e-mail to http://www.guilford.com.

REFERENCES AND RESOURCES FOR PROFESSIONALS

Aldwin, C., and Revenson, T. A. (1987). Does coping help? A reexamination of the relationship between coping and mental health. *Journal of Personality and Social Psychology, 53,* 337–348.

Bloom, S. (1997). *Creating sanctuary: Toward the evolution of sane societies.* New York: Routledge.

Briere, J. (1992). *Child abuse trauma: Theory and treatment of the lasting effects.* Newbury Park: Sage.

Burns, D. (1989). *The feeling good handbook.* New York: William Morrow & Co.

Carver, C., Scheier, M. F., and Weintraub, J. K. (1989). Assessing coping strategies: A theoretically based approach. *Journal of Personality and Social Psychology, 56.* 267–283.

Dattilio, F. M., and Freeman, A. (1994). *Cognitive-behavioral strategies in crisis intervention.* New York: Guilford Press.

Dunkel-Schetter, C., Feinstein, L. G., Taylor, S. E., and Falke, R. L. (1992). Patterns of coping with cancer. *Health Psychology, 11,* 79–87.

Figley, C. R. (Ed.). (1995). *Compassion fatigue: Secondary traumatic stress disorder from treating the traumatized.* New York: W.W. Norton.

Herman, J. L. (1992). *Trauma and recovery: The aftermath of violence from domestic abuse to political terror.* New York: Basic.

Janoff-Bulman, R. (1992). *Shattered assumptions: Toward a new psychology of trauma.* New York: Free Press.

Larson, D. G. (1993). *The helper's journey: Working with people facing grief, loss, and life-threatening illness.* Champaign, IL: Research Press.

Lazarus, R. S. (1993). Coping theory and research: Past, present, and future. *Psychosomatic Medicine, 55,* 234–247.

Lazarus, R. S., and Folkman, S. (1984). *Stress, appraisal, and coping.* New York: Springer.

Leehan, J., and Wilson, J. P. (1985). *Grown-up abused children.* Springfield, IL: Charles C. Thomas Publisher.

McCann, I. L., and Pearlman, L. A. (1990). *Psychological trauma and the adult survivor: Theory, therapy and transformation.* New York: Brunner/Mazel.

Padesky, C. A., and Greenberger, D. (1995). *A clinician's guide to mind over mood: A cognitive therapy treatment manual for clients.* New York: Guilford Press.

Pearlman, L. A., and Saakvitne, D. W. (1995). *Trauma and the therapist: Countertransference and vicarious traumatization in psychotherapy with incest survivors.* New York: W.W. Norton.

Resick, P. A., and Schnicke, M. K. (1993). *Cognitive processing therapy for rape victims: A treatment manual.* Newbury Park, CA: Sage.

Saakvitne, K. W., and Pearlman, (1996). *Transforming the pain: A workbook on vicarious traumatization.* New York: W.W. Norton.

Slaby, A. E. (1988). *Sixty ways to make stress work for you.* Summit, NJ: Psychiatric Institutes of America Press

Stamm, B. H. (Ed.). (1996). *Secondary traumatic stress: Self-care issues for clinicians, researchers and educators.* Lutherville, MD: Sidran Press.

Staub, E. (1989). *The roots of evil: The origins of genocide and other group violence.* Cambridge, UK: Cambridge University Press.

Van der Kolk, B. A., McFarlane, A. C., and Weisaeth, L. (Eds.). (1996). *Traumatic stress: The effects of overwhelming experience on mind, body and society.* New York: Guilford Press.

Williams, M. B., and Sommer, J. F. (Eds.). (1994). *Handbook of post-traumatic therapy.* Westport, CT: Greenwood Press.

Zinner, E., and Williams, M. B. (Eds.). (1998). *When a community weeps. Case studies in group survivorship.* Philadelphia, PA: Taylor & Francis.

INDEX

DEAR READER:

We hope you have found this workbook helpful. We welcome your feedback. Let us know your comments, ideas, or suggestions for future editions. You may forward comments to us, care of Guilford Press, at their mailing address (72 Spring Street, New York, New York 10012) or send them by e-mail (http://www.guilford.com).

THE AUTHORS

Order Form

Quantity Discounts Available for
Life After Trauma: A Workbook for Healing

To the Health Care Professional:

In order to make it easier for you to purchase multiple copies of this book for your clients, Guilford Publications is pleased to offer quantity discounts. In the order form below, simply multiply the discount price-per-book times the quantity you are ordering, and add 5% of your total order for shipping.

Quantity	Discount	*Price Per Book
1 book	—	$17.95
2-12 books	20% off list price	$14.36
13-24 books	30% off list price	$12.57
25+	33% off list price	$12.03

Guilford Publications, Inc.

Dept. 4R, 72 Spring Street, New York, NY 10012

CALL TOLL FREE (800) 365-7006
FAX: (212) 966-6708
E-MAIL: info@guilford.com
WEBSITE (secure online ordering): http://www.guilford.com

Name

Address   Rm./Apt. No.

City   State   Zip

(   )
Daytime Phone No.

☐ Please send me a complete Guilford Catalog, Cat. #CAT.

☐ Please do not put me on your mailing list

To order, please call the toll-free number above, order online at our website, or photocopy this coupon and mail or fax it today.

Qty	Cat. #	Title	*Price	Amount
	4R0239	**Life After Trauma**		

* * Shipping—For single-copy orders: In U.S., add $4.00; in Canada, add U.S.$7.50. For quantity orders, add 5% of total order.

* *Shipping	
Subtotal	
In NY and PA, add Sales Tax. In Canada, add G.S.T.	
TOTAL	

METHOD OF PAYMENT

☐ Check or Money Order Enclosed (U.S. Dollars only)

☐ Institutional P.O. Attached

BILL MY: ☐ MasterCard
          ☐ VISA
          ☐ American Express

Acct. #

Expiration Date

Month   Year

Signature (Required on Credit Card Orders)

All prices are in U.S. dollars. Prices are subject to change.